OXFORD

CW00554944

Mu

Oxford University Press makes no representation, express or implied, that the drug dosages in this book are correct. Readers must therefore always check the product information and clinical procedures with the most up-to-date published product information and data sheets provided by the manufacturers and the most recent codes of conduct and safety regulations. The authors and the publishers do not accept responsibility or legal liability for any errors in the text or for the misuse or misapplication of material in this work.

▶ Except where otherwise stated, drug doses and recommendations are for the non-pregnant adult who is not breast-feeding.

O N E L
OXFORD NEUROLOGY LIBRARY

Multiple Sclerosis

Neil Scolding

Burden Professor of Clinical Neurosciences,
University of Bristol and Consultant Neurologist,
North Bristol NHS Trust,
Bristol, UK

Alastair Wilkins

Consultant Senior Lecturer in Neurology,
University of Bristol;
Consultant Neurologist,
North Bristol NHS Trust
Bristol, UK

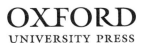

OXFORD
UNIVERSITY PRESS

OXFORD
UNIVERSITY PRESS

Great Clarendon Street, Oxford OX2 6DP,
United Kingdom

Oxford University Press is a department of the University of Oxford.
It furthers the University's objective of excellence in research, scholarship,
and education by publishing worldwide. Oxford is a registered trade mark of
Oxford University Press in the UK and in certain other countries

British Library Cataloguing in Publication Data

Data available

Library of Congress Cataloging in Publication Data

Data available

ISBN 978-0-19-960325-1

Printed in Great Britain by
Clays Ltd, St Ives plc

Contents

Preface

Neurology has a reputation for being a specialty dealing with rare, complex disorders, all of which are of completely unknown cause, and none of which are treatable. Multiple sclerosis is certainly complex, but no longer fulfils almost any other of these descriptions. It is one of the commonest neurological diseases; its causes are rapidly being dissected; a variety of disease-modifying treatments of varied efficacy (and safety) are now available and licensed, and more are being added year by year. Whilst a detailed picture of the fast-changing story of multiple sclerosis is available in a number of large and in depth monographs on the disease, we believe many clinicians would also welcome rapid pocket-access to the core clinical facts.

The function of this text is to provide such access to facts concerning the diagnosis and management of multiple sclerosis. We hope the information provided will assist the busy clinician in the diagnosis and treatment of the disease. The management strategies generally reflect those in current UK practice. Drug prescription and doses should be checked against local or national formularies and should be used in line with manufacturers' recommendations and licensing laws.

The authors would like to thank staff at the OUP for help in preparing the text. In addition we are indebted to our patients, colleagues and mentors for stimulating our interest in MS. Finally we would like to thank our families for their continuing support.

NJS
AW
2011

Symbols and abbreviations

ADEM	acute disseminated encephalomyelitis
ALD	adrenoleucodystrophy
ANCA	anti-neutrophil cytoplasmic antibody
APP	amyloid precursor protein
ARR	annualized relapse rate
BBB	blood-brain barrier
βIFN	beta interferons
BFID	benign focal inflammatory demyelination
CADASIL	cerebral autosomal dominant arteriopathy with subcortical infarcts and leukoencephalopathy
CBD	cannabidiol
CBT	cognitive-behavioural therapy
CIS	clinically isolated syndrome
CNP	central neuropathic pain
CNS	central nervous system
CSF	cerebrospinal fluid
DMT	disease modifying therapy
EAE	experimental allergic (or "autoimmune") encephalomyelitis
EBV	Epstein Barr Virus
EDSS	expanded disability status scale
ESR	erythrocyte sedimentation rate
GA	glatiramer acetate
GWAS	genome wide association screen
HIV	human immunodeficiency virus
HLA	Human Leukocyte Antigen
IRF8	interferon regulatory factor-8
ISC	intermittent self-catheterization
ITB	Intrathecal baclofen
LETM	longitudinally extensive transverse myelitis
LHON	Leber's hereditary optic neuropathy
LP	lumbar puncture

LVEF	left ventricular ejection fraction
MDEM	multi-phasic disseminated encephalomyelitis
MELAS	mitochondrial encephalopathy, lactic acidosis and stroke-like episodes
MHC	major histocompatability complex
MR	magnetic resonance
MRI	magnetic resonance imaging
MS	multiple sclerosis
NK	natural killer
NMO	neuromyelitis optica
OMIM	Online Mendelian Inheritance in Man
ON	optic neuritis
PAS	periodic acid-Schiff
PPMS	primary progressive multiple sclerosis
PVR	post-voiding residual volume
RRMS	relapsing and remitting multiple sclerosis
SBE	subacute bacterial endocarditis
SLE	systemic lupus erythematosus
SSRI	selective serotonin reuptake inhibitors
THC	tetrahydrocannabinol
TM	transverse myelitis
TN	trigeminal neuralgia
TNFRSF1A	tumour necrosis factor receptor superfamily member 1A
UTI	urinary tract infection
VLCFA	very long chain fatty acids

Chapter 1

Multiple sclerosis: an introduction

Multiple sclerosis (MS) affects around 400,000 in Europe, perhaps 2.5 million people worldwide. It costs the EU economy some €9 billion annually—mostly through the direct and indirect consequences of progressive disability in sufferers. MS has been known since its first description to cause such disability, notwithstanding the usual and defining relapsing-remitting initial course.

It is a disease of paradoxes and questions. Over 80% of MS patients develop progressive disability; and 40% of patients require a wheelchair within 10 years of diagnosis. A minority, however—those with so-called 'benign MS'—develops an illness which at onset appears identical clinically, radiologically, immunologically and neuropathologically, and yet these individuals acquire no significant disability over many decades of the disease. There is a significant genetic background, with over 30% concordance in identical twins; and yet individuals with MS in the same kindred may exhibit markedly different clinical phenotypes, and their disease pursue dramatically different courses. MS was amongst the first human diseases for which an experimental animal model was developed (80 years ago)—and yet despite continuous use of (and investment in) this model in different forms, there remains no cure now or even on any visible horizon, and the first 60 years or more of experimental modelling yielded not the slightest therapeutic dividend. There has been similarly a major worldwide investment in MR scanning of MS patients; and yet (very surprisingly to many non-neurologists) there remains no diagnostic test for MS—though 'real time' imaging of the disease has undoubtedly taught us an enormous amount about the behaviour and underlying features of MS. And finally, of course, the cause of MS remains unknown.

Each of these various aspects, and others, will be considered in the following, but it is perhaps worthwhile putting this brief account of where we are with MS into a context—how did we get here?

1.1 MS milestones

Multiple sclerosis (MS) has been familiar to neurologists since Charcot's description of the disease in 1868, during a hundred year

...

period (say, 1815–1915) when the foundations of classical clinical neurology were being laid in Europe, and the major neurological diseases—Parkinson's disease, motor neuron disease, Guillain-Barré syndrome, myasthenia gravis, Alzheimer's disease—were being delineated and described. Charcot recorded the relapsing-remitting nature of the disease, and the triad of features (nystagmus, intention tremor, and telegraphic speech) seen commonly in chronic cases.

Evidence for an immune and inflammatory basis underlying the disease came from pathological studies of MS in the first half of the 20th century, and from studies in the 1930's from Thomas Rivers and colleagues in the Rockefeller Institute. They described an MS-like illness in monkeys following the injection of rabbit brain extract— experimental allergic (or 'autoimmune') encephalomyelitis (EAE). This model (arguably far closer to acute disseminated encephalomy-elitis than to MS) has provided endless information about how the immune and nervous systems interact, whilst playing a limited role in the development of treatments.

The place of corticosteroids in treating MS relapses but not progressive disease was clarified in the 1960s, but it was another two decades before the first disease-modifying drugs developed, interferon-β and glatiramer acetate. The last decade has seen the introduction of therapeutic monoclonal antibodies in MS and the beginning of oral immune therapies, the delineation of NMO as an antibody-mediated disorder, and the emergence of a relationship between vitamin D and MS.

Other changes have come thick and fast over the last few years, and it is as ever difficult to gauge what place very recent devel-opments, let alone those which appear imminent, will ultimately occupy in any longer term narrative of MS. Will post-GWAS DNA studies finally allow genetics to make a real contribution to our understanding of MS? Will vitamin D prove to be the long specu-lated on environmental story factor? Or Epstein-Barr virus? Might the anti-aquaporin 4-NMO story, remarkable enough in itself, prove the key for unlocking a host of antibody specificities underlying further sub-types of MS? Will monoclonal antibodies reliably prevent not just relapses but secondary progression?

'Breakthroughs' in MS in the past have more often than not been ephemeral, rapidly contradicted or undermined by efforts to repeat experiments, or by larger, better executed studies, but it is still hard not to be optimistic about the short, medium and long term future in relation to this difficult disease. Before speculating briefly (Chapter 6) on what may be to come, we will first summarize the current position in relation to clinical, biological and therapeutic aspects of multiple sclerosis.

Chapter 2

The causes and mechanisms of multiple sclerosis

Key points

- Epidemiological studies of MS have been highly informative in guiding the search for aetiological factors in MS
- There are genetic influences governing disease susceptibility, the strongest of those being immune system genes
- No proven environmental 'cause' for MS has been discovered although several factors are thought to be important
- MS is immunologically driven and is likely to be initiated by autoimmune dysregulation
- A number of pathological processes occur in the central nervous system which are responsible for tissue damage and clinical manifestations of the disease.

3

Despite increasing understanding of disease mechanisms in MS and the increase in therapeutic options, the exact cause of the disease remains unknown. Most neurologists would now accept that a combination of genetic factors and environmental influences act to confer susceptibility to the disease. Downstream to the initiation of the disease, a number of immunological disturbances coupled to tissue and cell specific damage lead to the clinical manifestation of MS. The putative causes and downstream mechanisms will be discussed.

2.1 Epidemiology of MS

The epidemiology of MS has been studied extensively and this has led to improved understanding of the aetiology of the disease.

Of particular interest are the geographical variations in disease incidence, sex differences and age of onset data. Whilst these have given clues concerning the causes of MS, a unifying explanation of the epidemiology of the disease has so far not been forthcoming.

2.1.1 **Prevalence and geographical distribution of MS**

The incidence and prevalence of MS varies extensively between geographical locations. In addition, the incidence of MS is age dependent and is different in men and women. MS is prevalent in certain Northern European countries, such as the UK, Norway and Germany; and North America; with a prevalence in those areas of approximately 0.1% (100 per 100,000) of the population (see Figure 2.1). Some regions of individual countries, e.g. the Orkney Island in the UK or Sardinia in Italy, appear to have much higher prevalence rates than the rest of the country. The disease appears virtually absent in some populations, e.g. Chinese populations. In addition, in many Asian populations, MS is rare and when it occurs appears as an optico-spinal form of MS or as neuromyelitis optica. These differences in disease prevalence and phenotype are probably mostly determined by genetic factors in the different populations.

In some regions of the world MS prevalence increases with increasing latitude, such that regions closer to the equator appear to have lower rates than those further away. For instance, in the USA, the prevalence of MS in Florida is roughly half that of North Dakota. After controlling for ethnic origin, geographical latitude remains a risk factor for MS susceptibility. An attractive explanation to this effect is that reduced sunlight in more northern climates increases susceptibility to MS. However, this latitudinal gradient does not apply to all countries and there is evidence to suggest the latitude effect has reduced in recent times, emphasizing the notion that susceptibility to MS is likely to be multifactorial.

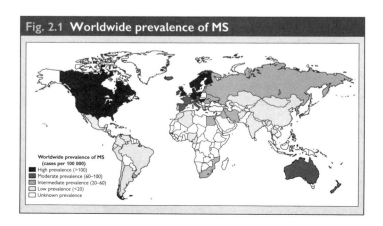

Fig. 2.1 **Worldwide prevalence of MS**

Worldwide prevalence of MS
(cases per 100 000)
- High prevalence (>100)
- Moderate prevalence (60–100)
- Intermediate prevalence (20–60)
- Low prevalence (<20)
- Unknown prevalence

2.1.2 **Sex and age at disease onset**

The female to male ratio of MS incidence is approaching 3:1 irrespective of ethnicity. Age of onset of MS does however appear to influence sex ratios since, for instance, MS presents in the fifth decade in a more even sex ratio, whereas in paediatric populations the female to male ratio may be as high as 3:1. The reason for the differences in incidence between sexes is unknown. Genome wide studies have not implicated the sex chromosomes as having any susceptibility or protective role.

Age at presentation of MS shows peak incidence of the disease in the 4th decade of life (between the age of 30 and 40). The disease remains rare at the extremes of life, although approximately 5% of all MS cases present in childhood. The incidence of MS drops significantly after the age of 50 and is extremely rarely diagnosed in those over the age of 70 (see Figure 2.2).

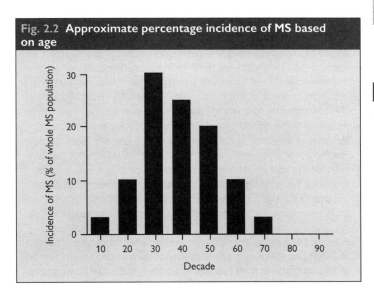

Fig. 2.2 Approximate percentage incidence of MS based on age

Incidence of MS (% of whole MS population) vs *Decade*

2.1.3 **Migration and ethnicity**

Ethnicity plays an important role in MS susceptibility, reflecting genetic influences independent of shared environmental risk factors. For instance, in Australia and New Zealand MS is rarely diagnosed in Aborigines or Maoris but occurs commonly in those of Caucasian origin. Similarly, after controlling for confounding factors, African American men have a lower risk of MS than white American men by approximately 40%.

In order to dissect out genetic and environmental factors, migration studies between geographical areas of high and low risk have been informative. The majority of migrant studies suggest that the migrant's country of birth appears to be a major influence on risk of developing MS. Furthermore, age at migration appears to have an important effect, such that those who migrate before adolescence have an MS risk that approaches the risk of their adopted country, whereas those who migrate later in life probably keep the risk similar to that of their country of origin. This has given rise to the concept that an environmental factor (such as an infection) may act in a crucial time period to expose the risk of MS. Potential aetiological agents for MS are discussed.

2.1.4 **Other factors governing MS incidence**
Most researchers would now agree that there is an underlying genetic susceptibility risk for MS which is modulated by environmental risk factors, most likely occurring in a critical time window. Several other epidemiological observations relating to MS risk have also been made:

- *Month of birth*: interestingly in the Northern hemisphere, significantly more people with MS are born in April or May than are born in November. This 'month of birth' phenomenon suggests a seasonably variable risk factor and one which potentially acts in the antenatal or neonatal period
- *Parent of origin effects*: 'parent of origin' studies are used to determine whether specific genetic risks are more likely to be conferred from an individual's mother or father. In MS, there is evidence to suggest a maternal parent of origin effect, since maternal half-siblings of patients with MS (i.e. those that share a mother but have a different father) have roughly double the risk of MS compared with paternal half-siblings. The reason for this observation remains unknown, but epigenetic mechanisms (changes in gene expression by mechanisms other than changes in DNA sequence, e.g. DNA methylation and chromatin remodelling) interacting with MS susceptibility genes may play a part.

2.1.5 **Epidemiology of the disease course**
At the time of diagnosis of MS or when MS has been considered (e.g. first inflammatory event), it is important to give patients some idea concerning the likely course of the disease. Epidemiological studies have been helpful in determining data on disease course on a population basis. Predominantly these studies have been conducted by interrogating MS databases which have gathered information on such things as relapses and disability scores. It is worth emphasizing to patients that significant individual variation occurs in MS and predicting accurately the future course of the disease is not possible.

Certain useful figures can be gleaned from the studies assessing the impact of MS over time.

- *Conversion of clinically isolated syndrome to clinically definite MS*: The majority of those developing MS will initially present with a clinically isolated syndrome (CIS). However, not all those with CIS will go on to develop MS. The development of clinically definite MS occurs in approximately two-thirds of those with CIS over a period of 20 years
- *Relapse rates in RRMS*: The annualized relapse rate (ARR) in patients with RRMS is of the order of 0.4 (i.e. the average number of relapses per year). Treatment trials generally report higher rates in their placebo arms which probably reflect the inclusion criteria for trials which study patients with higher numbers of relapses. Relapses are often noted to occur more frequently early in the disease course and usually reduce in frequency in chronic disease. Evidence suggests that relapse rates may be higher in paediatric populations compared to adults
- *Time to disability milestones*: Defining the onset of disease progression in individual patients is difficult and is often noted in retrospect. However, patients will often wish to know likely prognosis concerning mobility over their lifetime. The number of years to progress through disability milestones is highly variable and age at presentation and the type of disease onset (RRMS vs. PPMS) are key factors. For instance those presenting with a progressive onset will reach disability milestones more quickly and those presenting at a later age will, in general, progress through disability milestones more quickly. Epidemiological data on patient populations has suggested that a patient presenting with MS in their 30s might take approximately 18 years to needing to walk with unilateral walking aid (stick/cane) and 25 years to require a wheelchair. It should be emphasized that these are population figures and the progress of an individual may be very different.

2.2 **Causes of MS**

The cause of MS remains unknown. As with many common disorders, it is likely that a combination of genetic and environmental influences is involved in both the pathogenesis of the disorder and in determining the course of the disease. This latter aspect, that is understanding why some people with MS have a fairly benign course whilst others have a more severe, progressive illness, remains a huge challenge to researchers. In recent years, improved understanding of genetic and environmental factors in MS has occurred which, in time, will hopefully translate into better therapies for the disease. Furthermore, advances in understanding disease heterogeneity which has led to separating out distinct disease entities, such as neuromyelitis optica, will help in further delineating the causes of MS.

2.2.1 **Genetics of MS**

The search for genes underlying the pathogenesis of MS has been active for over 40 years. Although MS is not a pure Mendelian genetic disorder, epidemiological studies demonstrated many years ago that there are genetic influences regulating the specific risk of acquiring the disease in individuals. In recent years the number of genes which have been implicated in disease susceptibility has grown significantly and there is now a clearer understanding of which genetic substrates appear to be associated with development of the disease. Whilst each individual gene may play a small role in disease susceptibility, it is hoped that by understanding the particular combinations of genetic influences that researchers will be able to better understand the pathogenesis of the disease and also design rational disease-modifying drugs. In keeping with many common diseases complex genetic effects, environmental influences and disease heterogeneity mean that MS is characterized by modest heritability. It is unlikely that advances in genetic profiling will be able, in the near future, to provide a lifetime risk of MS to an individual.

2.2.1.1 Familial clustering

It is relatively common for patients with MS to report a family history of the disease and patients will often ask the risk to relatives. Between 15–20% of patients with MS have a family history, a rate higher than might be expected by chance. Twin studies have shown that monozygotic twins have a much higher concordance rate of MS (approximately 30%) than dizygotic twins (approximately 5%), indicating a significant genetic aetiology for MS. A non-twin sibling of a patient with MS has a roughly 3% risk of acquiring the disease, compared to a background prevalence (in temperate regions) of 0.1%. The sibling recurrence risk ratio (λ_s) in MS is approximately 15–20 (which is similar to that of type-1 diabetes mellitus in Caucasian populations). Second and third degree relatives of patients with MS are also at increased risk of MS, albeit at lower levels, again indicating some degree of familial susceptibility, distinct from shared environmental factors. Identifying susceptibility genes and delineating genetic influences from environmental risk factors has been the subject of intense research.

2.2.1.2 Human Leukocyte Antigens

MS is characterized by complex genetic effects and identifying susceptibility genes has proved difficult. In the main, this is likely due to the modest effect of individual genes and the significant degree of genetic variation in the human population. The number of susceptibility genes in MS is not known, but studies have suggested that a large number of genes, each with modest genetic effects are responsible for the heritability of MS.

The first identified genetic association with MS was the Human Leukocyte Antigen (HLA) region on chromosome 6 which remains the most potent genetic susceptibility factor for MS identified. HLA genes (within the major histocompatability complex (MHC)) are involved in the response to pathogens, specifically in orchestrating antigen presentation to immune cells, immune recognition of 'self' from 'non-self' and in orchestrating cytokine release and complement activation. The involvement of HLA genes in MS, a disease characterized by immunological disturbances, is not unexpected. Indeed, the hypothesis that modulation of antigen presentation leading to alterations in immunological recognition of self-antigens is an attractive aetiological theory.

The HLA region is characterized by high degrees of polymorphism and particular alleles have been associated with susceptibility to MS. Most notably, the DRB1*1501 allele has been most closely associated and has been replicated in virtually all populations, particularly those of Northern European ancestry. Nonetheless, the majority of those carrying the DRB1*1501 allele will not go on to develop MS and approximately 45% of patients with MS do not harbour the allele, emphasizing the complexity of genetic susceptibility. Overall, epistatic interactions between HLA alleles are thought to be responsible for approximately 50% of the genetic risk of MS.

2.2.1.3 Newer susceptibility genes
Finding non-HLA susceptibility genes for MS has proved challenging and has required large sample numbers in order to provide sufficient power to detect very modest genetic effects of individual genes. However, technological advances and the human genome project have led to an exponential growth in the understanding of genetics of complex diseases. Several powerful genome-wide association studies have now been reported and have yielded promising non-HLA candidate genes. At the time of writing, the list of MS susceptibility genes is growing, although many await further verification. Of interest, single nucleotide polymorphisms conferring susceptibility to MS in two interleukin receptor genes, IL7R and IL2RA, have been implicated, highlighting the importance in the genetic regulation of the immune response in the aetiology of the disease. Other recently discovered genes with modest susceptibility effects include CD58, CD6, interferon regulatory factor-8 (IRF8) and tumour necrosis factor receptor superfamily member 1A (TNFRSF1A), all of which have regulatory roles in the generation and propagation of inflammatory responses. The Online Mendelian Inheritance in Man (OMIM)

section of the NCBI website has up to date information on genetic susceptibility studies in MS (http://www.ncbi.nlm.nih.gov/omim/126200).

2.2.1.4 Future genetic studies

Understanding how susceptibility genes interact to confer the risk of MS to an individual remains a challenge for the coming years. Also trying to determine how genetic factors influence disease course is of major interest. For instance, questions that arise include: are there specific genetic variations which underlie the PPMS phenotype? Are there genetic cues which influence early disease progression? Is relapse frequency determined by genetic factors?

In a similar way, understanding how genetic influences interact with environmental factors will allow for a much better understanding of disease pathogenesis. Recently, HLA-DRB1*1501 expression has been shown to be regulated by vitamin D, suggesting a possible link between environmental and genetic factors in MS.

Box 2.1 Summary of genetic factors involved in MS

Genetic factors and MS

- Family studies have demonstrated a significant genetic basis for MS susceptibility
- HLA genes, specifically DRB1, have the strongest genetic influence on disease susceptibility
- Many other susceptibility genes are being identified, although the influence of individual non-HLA genes is individually small
- Understanding interactions of susceptibility genes with each other and with environmental influences will lead to a greater understanding of the aetiology of MS.

2.2.2 **Environmental factors and MS**

Research into MS has highlighted a number of environmental factors with a potential association to MS onset. At the present time, the strongest evidence has accumulated for two agents with a potential link to MS pathogenesis- Epstein Barr Virus (EBV) and vitamin D, though a consensus is yet to be achieved in relation to either.

2.2.2.1 EBV

EBV is a DNA virus of the herpes family which causes infectious mononucleosis and has been linked to the pathogenesis of some cancers. There is also evidence that it is linked with the pathogenesis of several autoimmune diseases including systemic lupus erythematosus, dermatomyositis and rheumatoid arthritis. Recent evidence has suggested the virus may also be involved in the immunopathogenesis of MS. Over 90% of the general adult population has been infected at some time with EBV, implying that if EBV is implicated there must be other modifiable factors. EBV infection at an early age is usually asymptomatic, whereas infection in adolescence or adulthood may lead to infectious mononucleosis. Nearly all adult patients with MS (>99%) have been infected at some time with EBV, with the incidence of MS being 2–3 fold higher in those who have had infectious mononucleosis compared to those who have not. Serological studies have shown that those with a higher titre of anti-EBV antibodies have a higher risk of developing MS, compared to those with lower titres. EBV is known to infect B lymphocytes and may immortalize them into long-lived memory B cells, capable of prolonged survival in the peripheral circulation. Interestingly, in the years before development of the disease, plasma levels of EBV nuclear antigen-1 (EBNA1) increase over time before clinical onset of MS. Attempts to detect EBV infection within the central nervous system of patients with MS using post mortem pathological analysis has led to some conflicting results, although some researchers have suggested there may be EBV latency within B cells residing in the brain. There is no evidence for disease-specific intrathecal synthesis of anti-EBV antibodies in MS.

Theories relating to the mechanisms by which EBV is implicated in MS pathogenesis include antigenic mimicry, B-cell clone immortalization, and dysregulation of cytotoxic T-cells against EBV-infected B cells. Whether EBV has its major effect peripherally, i.e. by inducing immune changes within circulating peripheral lymphocytes, or centrally, i.e. through direct central nervous system immune dysregulation, is not clear. If more evidence accumulates to implicate EBV in MS aetiology, the next step will be to determine whether treatment with anti-EBV therapies may help in the acute stages of the disease. Preliminary trials with valacyclovir or alacyclovir have been inconclusive. Furthermore, whether reduction of paediatric infection with EBV via vaccination programmes would be warranted, would raise major public health questions, since the consequences of eliminating infection by such a common virus at a population level are unknown.

2.2.2.2 Vitamin D and sunlight exposure

The observations relating to geographical latitude and MS incidence discussed could potentially be explained by sunlight exposure and associated vitamin D status. Vitamin D_3 (colecalciferol) is made in the skin by the action of ultraviolet (B) light on 7-dehydrocholesterol. The circulating form of vitamin D is 25-hydroxyvitamin D. There is some evidence that vitamin D levels may influence MS, particularly relapse occurrence.

In keeping with the latitude data, epidemiological studies have suggested that an inverse relationship between past sunlight exposure and MS susceptibility exists. Whether vitamin D itself mediates this sunlight effect is not clear. However, recent case control studies have suggested a high serum concentration of 25-hydroxyvitamin D is associated with low risk of MS. Furthermore, low levels of 25-hydroxyvitamin D are found in RRMS (compared to healthy control), particularly in the period prior to relapse. These observations provide a rationale for further research on vitamin D and MS, although the evidence does remain circumstantial. In order to determine precisely the effect of vitamin D on MS susceptibility and relapse rates, clinical trials are required. Existing trials of vitamin supplementation have not been able to determine whether vitamin D has a protective effect, but further trials are in progress. The role of vitamin D in the immune system is also attracting much interest in relation to other autoimmune diseases.

2.2.2.3 Other possible environmental factors

In keeping with the likely multi-factorial aetiology of MS, many other putative environmental triggers have been postulated. It remains possible that, given a susceptible genetic background, a number of environmental stimuli may trigger the disease. Indeed a variety of genotypes may interact with their own specific environmental triggers to produce the same phenotype of disease, although dissecting out these interactions will prove hugely challenging. Other environmental factors that may be important in the pathogenesis of MS include:

- *Smoking*: epidemiological studies have suggested that smoking cigarettes infers a modest increased risk of MS (Odds Ratio approximately 1.5)

- *Other infections*: in clinical practice relapses are often noted to occur shortly after or during intercurrent infections. Whilst this may reflect changes in generic immune networks rather than specific pathogen induced auto-immunity, the search for viral or bacterial agents which may increase susceptibility to MS or induce relapses continues. However, some evidence points to exposure to infectious triggers prior to the onset of adolescence may be key to future development of MS

- *Vaccinations*: whether vaccinations may induce disease relapses has been the subject of a number of studies. The conclusion of most studies has been that vaccination (with common vaccines including seasonal influenza vaccine) does not appear to increase the short-term risk of relapse in multiple sclerosis. It is also interesting to note that since the introduction of widespread childhood vaccination programmes in Western countries the incidence of MS has not dropped, even though the early vaccination population has gone well into the susceptible age for the disease

- *Trauma:* patients often report antecedent trauma (e.g. head injury) prior to onset of MS diagnosis or relapse. It is often hard to determine whether this represents reporting bias or whether immunological changes which have been documented to occur in trauma have some influence on MS.

2.3 Mechanisms of MS

MS is typically characterized by clinical relapses representing damage or disturbance in function to specific parts of the central nervous system. These areas of damage are disseminated in time and space. Furthermore many patients have, either in addition or as the sole manifestation of the disease, progressive neurological deterioration. How can these seemingly disparate observations be tied together? And does MS represent one disease process or a number and can the pathological events of MS be tied together?

In keeping with knowledge of the causes of MS, the precise mechanistic cascade of the disease is not fully understood. It is generally accepted that a primary immunological event drives the disease with subsequent CNS tissue injury. Immunological mechanisms and pathological processes will be reviewed in brief.

2.3.1 Immunology of MS

MS is classically thought of as a T cell-dependent process associated with macrophage-mediated demyelination driven by a myelin-specific autoantigen. It is likely that peripheral immunological activation (via antigen(s) as yet undetermined) occurs outside of the nervous system with subsequent spread into the CNS via blood-brain barrier breakdown. Further amplification of the immune/inflammatory response then occurs within the CNS with recruitment of macrophages and CNS microglia. Both cellular (cytotoxic) processes and release of soluble factors by inflammatory cells are thought to mediate CNS tissue damage.

2.3.1.1 Autoimmune hypothesis of MS

Based upon observations in experimental models of MS (mostly experimental autoimmune encephalomyelitis; EAE), the autoimmune hypothesis of MS induction has been widely postulated. This hypothesis suggests that lymphocytes may be activated by foreign antigen(s) (probably a pathogen) with subsequent cellular proliferation. Following CNS entry, a process of molecular mimicry (whereby immune cells activated by foreign antigen abnormally recognize a similar self-antigen in the CNS) sets up an autoimmune process. The identities of the foreign antigen or the autoantigen are unknown, but myelin components seem likely to be autoantigenic targets. Indeed, myelin-antigen specific T cells can be isolated from peripheral blood lymphocytes of MS patients. The autoimmune hypothesis of MS implies a failure of innate tolerance mechanisms which should normally operate to protect against autoimmunity.

2.3.1.2 T lymphocyte driven autoimmunity

T lymphocytes play an important role in the generation and propagation of immune changes in MS. The precise immunological driver for MS has been the subject of intense debate for a number of years. Many of the putative immunological mechanisms derive from studies in EAE, in which CD4+ T cells polarized to T_h (T-helper; and specifically T_h1) phenotype induce much of the immunological damage. CD4+ T_h lymphocytes are classically divided into a number of further subtypes dependent on their cytokine expression profile and influence on effector cells (see Figure 2.3).

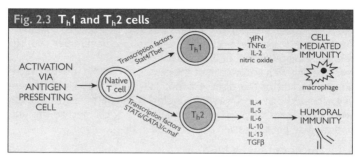

Fig. 2.3 **T_h1 and T_h2 cells**

Dysregulated T_h1 responses are thought to be responsible for the organ specific autoimmunity of MS through actions of cytokines such as γIFN. CD4+ T_h cells are highly prominent cells within active MS lesions. Furthermore, the cytokine profile classically associated with T_h1 cells, γIFN, TNFα and IL-2, are found in acute lesions and these cytokines (as well as mRNA transcripts of these cytokines) can be detected in tissue and CSF derived from patients with MS. T_h1 cells also activate macrophages and microglia, which are prominent in inflammatory infiltrates. The exact distinction between T_h1 and T_h2 cells may, however, not be as distinct as in rodent models and in recent years it has become clear that the immunological interplay is much more complicated than first thought.

MHC class 1-restricted, CD8+ T cells are also prominent in active MS lesions. It is possible that these cells are primarily responsible for acute axonal damage within lesions. Previously unknown contributors to the disease process in MS include T_h17 cells (producing IL-17). mRNA encoding IL-17 has been detected at high levels in CSF, blood and in brain tissue of patients with MS. A further class of T cells called T-reg (FOXp3+ cells) are involved in the process of tolerance and immunosuppression. Defining further how T-reg cells inhibit T_h1 or T_h17 cells may be a major target for therapeutic intervention. Other effector populations include CD56+ natural killer (NK) cells, invariant NK cells and possibly stem cells. The further processes of tissue damage secondary to immune activation will be discussed.

2.3.1.3 B cells and MS

There is also evidence for the role of humoral immunity in MS. Pathological specimens have shown immunoglobulin and complement in degenerating myelin sheaths and the occurrence of plasma cells in plaques. Lymphoid follicles, in which B cell selection occurs, are found within the CNS of patients with MS and their presence may be indicative of a more severe disease. Furthermore, oligoclonal bands, which represent intrathecal antibody synthesis, are found in the majority of MS cases. It is not clear against which molecules these antibodies are directed and there is no real evidence to suggest they are anti-myelin. The precise role of B cells in the disease is unknown. B cells may act as antigen presenting cells and it is possible that they are involved in disease initiation and maintenance.

2.3.1.4 Implications for therapy

An understanding of the immunological processes occurring in MS has been crucial in developing therapies for the disease, while the incomplete nature of this understanding helps explain unexpected outcomes of a number of experimental clinical trials. A number of disease-modifying therapies are available (see Chapter 5) which target the immune system. Monoclonal antibody therapies which can address specific aspects of immune function are likely to have a very important role in the future. Trials have shown that modifying lymphocyte numbers (e.g. alemtuzumab) or their entry into the CNS (e.g. natalizumab) can impact significantly on disease activity. Trials have also demonstrated that such immune modulations are not without their problems and different immunologically-mediated diseases may emerge (see Chapter 5). In addition other trials have shown that targeting of specific aspects of the immune system may not always be helpful and may indeed be harmful. As an example, trials of TNFα-blocking agents in MS demonstrated worsening of disease activity. Further understanding of the toxic and protective qualities of the immune system in MS need to be undertaken in order to develop further highly specific and safe agents for therapeutic use.

2.3.2 Pathology of MS

Examination of post-mortem tissue in patients who have suffered with MS during their lifetime can be very useful in delineating mechanisms of disease. MS tissue is characterized by lesions corresponding to those seen on MRI ante-mortem. In addition a number of more diffuse changes throughout the nervous system are seen. Lesions often demonstrate varying degrees of inflammatory activity. Changes in immune cells, oligodendrocytes and their myelin, astrocytes, and axons are commonly seen reflecting a number of pathological processes in the disease. Whilst post mortem analysis is highly useful in determining putative disease mechanisms, tissue analysed in this way may only reflect a 'snap shot' of the disease, and usually one which has been progressing or active over a number of years. Tissue from patients who have died a short period of time after diagnosis, those with fulminant disease or those who have had brain biopsies also provide useful information.

Precise pathways in MS pathogenesis and specifically understanding the temporal sequence of events are not fully worked out, although knowledge concerning aspects of disease pathology is extensive. A schematic diagram of the putative cascade of events associated with MS pathology is shown (see Figure 2.4).

Fig. 2.4 Schematic diagram of pathological processes in MS

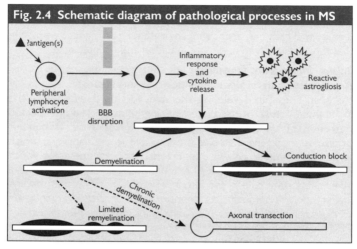

The classic hallmark of MS pathology is the sclerotic plaque, which is characterized by inflammation, demyelination, oligodendrocyte depletion, astrocytosis and axonal injury. MS plaques can be further classified by the degree of inflammatory activity and are often termed active or acute; chronic active; and inactive.

The events relating to generation of the sclerotic plaque will be discussed in more detail. Initial events which are thought to be critical in the generation of immunological disturbances of MS are discussed.

2.3.2.1 Blood brain barrier disruption

Disruption in the integrity of endothelial cell tight junctions occurs as an early feature of MS and breakdown of the blood-brain barrier (BBB) is thought to be an initiating factor in the process of CNS inflammation occurring in MS. Neuroimaging studies have been useful in providing an *in vivo* correlate of this phenomenon, since enhancement of lesions with gadolinium reflects BBB permeability. The precise cause of BBB disruption is unknown, but release of cytokines and vasoactive molecules by inflammatory cells within the perivascular space are likely mechanisms. Indeed lymphocytes and monocytes/macrophages within perivascular cell cuffs are an early feature of MS lesions. It is thought that disruptions of perivascular spaces are crucial processes in connecting peripheral immune activation with CNS disease.

2.3.2.2 Acute inflammation

Acute inflammatory cell infiltrate is a cardinal feature of MS pathology. T lymphocytes are abundant in active lesions of MS and thought to be predominantly responsible for initiating cytokine-mediated demyelination. CD4+ T lymphocytes are central to lesion formation, but equally CD8+ lymphocytes are abundant. B-lymphocytes and plasma cells are generally less numerous than T-cells. Macrophages, however, are the most numerous cells within active lesions, and are primarily involved in the process of myelin phagocytosis. Macrophages arise either from attracted circulating monocytes or are derived from resident CNS microglial populations.

2.3.2.3 Myelin injury and demyelination

Demyelinated plaques within white matter are the hallmark of MS (see Figure 2.5). Myelin is produced by oligodendrocytes within the CNS and ensheaths axons, allowing for rapid saltatory conduction. Failure or reduction in axonal action potential propagation is the likely substrate for the majority of neurological symptoms in early disease or during relapse. This phenomenon, however, does not depend solely on loss of myelin, since conduction block may occur in the absence of frank demyelination. Conduction block occurs through a variety of soluble mediators impairing normal action potential propagation and is reversible, suggesting an explanation for remission following resolution of inflammation.

Determining whether there is a specific antigen-mediated immune process responsible for oligodendrocyte injury and demyelination has proved difficult in MS, although a variety of putative myelin and non-myelin autoantigens have been proposed. Pathological specimens from acute lesions and post mortem analysis have suggested that there may be a number of different mechanistic subtypes responsible for demyelination including macrophage-associated demyelination; antibody/complement-mediated demyelination; distal 'dying-back' oligodendrocyte loss; and primary oligodendrocyte apoptosis. The relevance of these observations and the implications for disease heterogeneity are not clear.

Microglia, recruited and activated in the inflammatory milieu, undoubtedly play a role in oligodendrocyte and myelin injury via release of reactive oxygen and nitrogen species. Nitric oxide is a potent cytotoxic agent within the CNS and there is significant evidence for its role in MS.

B cells, which under normal conditions are not found in CNS parenchyma, are numerous in early MS lesions. Clonal proliferation

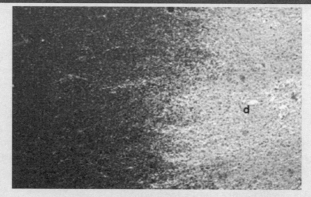

Fig. 2.5 Demyelination in brain white matter of patient with MS. Stained for Myelin Basic Protein (MBP); d represents area of demyelinated white matter

Picture courtesy of Dr. E. Gray, MS Labs, Frenchay Hospital; Tissue provided by MS Society of Great Britain and Northern Ireland Tissue Bank

of B cells occurs in the intrathecal compartment associated with restricted immunoglobulin banding patterns (oligoclonal bands), an important diagnostic feature of MS. Whether specific B cell clonal proliferation and antibody production drives myelin injury is unknown, although there is a wealth of information from experimental animal studies of demyelination to show that, in principle, this is a possible pathological mechanism. Similarly the precise role of T cells in oligodendrocyte injury is unknown, yet it seems likely that multiple T cell populations may specifically target and injure oligodendrocytes.

Remyelination does occur in MS lesions and may be extensive. When remyelination occurs, the sheath is generally thinner with a reduced internodal distance. However, chronic plaques are characterized by persistent demyelination. Understanding why remyelination fails in MS is the subject of intense research, since overcoming this block is a target for therapeutic intervention. Chronic inflammation causing persistent myelin injury, glial scarring, failure of maturation of oligodendrocyte precursor cells and changes to the extracellular matrix in lesions are likely to contribute. In addition, adult axons express molecules which inhibit myelin formation which is probably a key factor in the failure of remyelination.

2.3.2.4 Astrocytosis

Normal astrocyte structure and function may be perturbed in MS lesions. Hypertrophic astrocytes are commonly seen, particularly surrounding early lesions. Whether the astrocyte response is purely reactive or whether it serves some form of protective function is unknown.

2.3.2.5 Axonal injury

Axonal injury and loss is noted throughout the course of the disease. Pathologically disruptions in axonal transport and axonal structure are noted. Accumulations of amyloid precursor protein (APP) along the length of axons represents disruption in fast axonal transport and changes in neurofilament phosphorylation state are used to determine structural problems within the axon (see Figure 2.6). Furthermore, axonal spheroids represent transected axons.

Fig. 2.6 Axonal changes in white matter of patient with MS. Staining for non-phosphorylated neurofilament (SMI32)

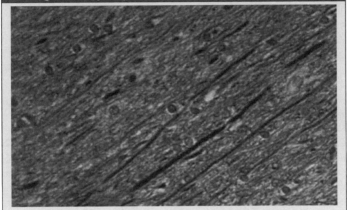

Picture courtesy of Dr. E. Gray, MS Labs, Frenchay Hospital; Tissue provided by MS Society of Great Britain and Northern Ireland Tissue Bank

Axonal injury appears most prevalent in acute inflammatory lesions and may be caused by direct inflammatory/immunological attack on axons. Axonal injury is also noted in chronic active and inactive lesions. Many researchers have postulated that post-inflammatory 'drop-out' of axons may occur in the chronic progressive phases of MS due to the loss of the normal supporting environment of the CNS. Indeed myelin itself seems to maintain axons in the long term and demyelination renders axons more susceptible to damage.

2.3.2.6 Grey matter disease

Traditionally MS is considered a disease of white matter. However, significant numbers of plaques occur within or extend into the grey matter (Figure 2.7). Conventional MRI imaging is poor at determining grey matter lesions in vivo, which, perhaps, explains the relative paucity of research on grey matter lesions compared to white matter.

Some of the more 'cortical' clinical features, such as cognitive impairment and epilepsy, seen in chronic progressive disease may be the correlate of chronic grey matter disease.

Fig. 2.7 Demyelination in brain white matter extending into the grey matter of patient with MS. Stained for Myelin Basic Protein (MBP); c represents cortical grey matter; arrows represent the edges of the plaque

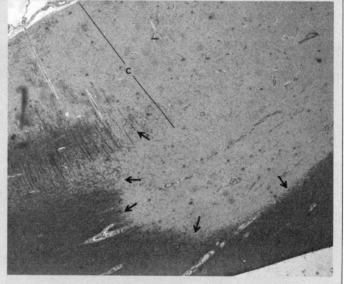

Picture courtesy of Dr. E. Gray, MS Labs, Frenchay Hospital; Tissue provided by MS Society of Great Britain and Northern Ireland Tissue Bank

Suggested reading

Ascherio A. and Munger K.L. (2010) Epstein-barr virus infection and multiple sclerosis: a review. *J Neuroimmune Pharmacol* **5**(3): 271–7.

Ascherio A., Munger K.L and Simon K.C. (2010) Vitamin D and multiple sclerosis. *Lancet Neurol*, **9**(6): 599–612.

Bennett J.L. and Stuve O. (2009) Update on inflammation, neurodegeneration, and immunoregulation in multiple sclerosis: therapeutic implications. *Clin Neuropharmacol* **32**(3): 121–32.

Confavreux C., et al. (2001) Vaccinations and the risk of relapse in multiple sclerosis. Vaccines in Multiple Sclerosis Study Group. *N Engl J Med* **344**(5): 319–26.

Oksenberg J.R., et al. (2008) The genetics of multiple sclerosis: SNPs to pathways to pathogenesis. *Nat Rev Genet* **9**(7): 516–26.

Sawcer S. (2008) The complex genetics of multiple sclerosis: pitfalls and prospects. *Brain* **131**(Pt 12): 3118–31.

Sobel R. and Moore G.R.W. (2009) Demyelinating diseases. *Greenfield's Neuropathology* (ed. Love, Louis, Ellison), pp. 1513–1608.

Chapter 3

Clinical presentations and disease course of multiple sclerosis

> **Key points**
> - MS commonly presents with sub-acutely deteriorating focal neurological symptoms and signs—the classical relapsing-remitting course
> - Around 10% of patients present with slowly progressive neurological problems—primary progressive MS
> - progressive and relapsing components of MS are clinically and pathologically quite different
> - Devic's disease, or neuromyelitis, is associated with anti-aquaporin 4 antibodies and a distinct clinical and radiological phenotype
> - Acute disseminated encephalomyelitis (ADEM) can sometimes resemble MS, but carries a more serious immediate risk, though it does not pursue a chronic progressive course in survivors of the acute illness.

3.1 Common clinical presentations of MS

MS remains predominantly a clinical diagnosis, and the clinical phenomenology, as with so many neurological diseases, is therefore vital. A classical patient might be a female (the steadily increasing female:male ratio, now well beyond the conventionally mentioned 2:1, remains unexplained) in her third or fourth decade, presenting with an 'attack' or inflammatory event (often called a relapse, though the term should be restricted to the second and subsequent events). Such attacks may be best termed *isolated demyelinating syndromes* or *focal inflammatory demyelination*.

The onset of attacks follows the typical course of inflammatory neurological disease, with progression over days to a week or so. Unlike the great majority of other inflammation-based disorders, however, MS events then spontaneously plateau (for a few days) before steadily improving over a period of a few weeks—usually back to normal, though a residual deficit is not uncommon.

(More paroxysmal clinical disturbances can also occur in MS, lasting minutes to hours; these are commonly unpleasant positive sensory phenomena or focal motor attacks—tonic spasms—and reflect electrophysiological excitement in previously damaged areas rather than new inflammatory lesions. Classical sensory disturbances, including Lhermitte's symptom (an 'electric shock' sensation triggered by flexing the neck) and Uhthoff's phenomenon (worsening of neurological symptoms with increased body temperature) are comparable. None 'count' as relapses, which must by definition last over 24 hours.)

A clinical diagnosis of multiple sclerosis may be apparent when two inflammatory events, affecting different parts of the central nervous system, occur. Not all individuals with one attack will develop a second; some patients remain permanently free of further events. There must be a stipulated 30 days between the onset of event 1 and event 2 for them to be regarded as 'separated in time'.

Although any part of the CNS may be affected by attacks, certain pathways are more vulnerable, for example:

- Acute *optic neuritis* typically presents with monocular visual loss and pain worse on eye movement. It is the initial experience of 14–23% MS patients
- *Corticospinal tract involvement* occurs with the initial attack in 32–41% patients. Spinal cord lesions are typically partial not complete, and bladder involvement common
- Brain stem disturbances, causing ataxia, diplopia, and/or long tract signs, can occur.

In all such cases, similar clinical events can occur in entirely unrelated disorders (see Chapter 4), and an episode of *focal inflammatory demyelination* cannot necessarily be assumed.

3.2 **Progressive disease**

The great majority—85–90%—of patients with multiple sclerosis commence their disease course with episodes of focal inflammatory demyelination, and with good recovery from each attack. On *average*, the interval between episodes might be 12–18 months, but this varies greatly.

However, after a period which can vary from a very few years to several decades, an entirely different clinical phenomenon emerges in most patients, namely that of progressive disability. There may be day-to-day fluctuation, but little persistent change over days, weeks or even months, but season by season, year by year, there is relentlessly advancing disability. (In some patients, relapses may also occur, complicating the clinical picture, but in most these become less frequent.)

Again, most parts of the CNS can be affected, but again, certain pathways and areas are more likely to be affected—typically a spastic paraparesis develops, with prominent bladder disturbance (often with bowel and sexual dysfunction). Strength tends to be retained in the upper limbs, but function if anything more dramatically reduced by an often severe proximal bilateral arm tremor. Brain stem/cerebellar damage is also responsible for the characteristic *internuclear ophthalmoplegia* also seen in chronic progressive MS. Severe fatigue and, later, cognitive impairment are also common.

Inexplicably, around 10% of patients never develop progressive problems—so-called *benign* MS. Others by contrast never have attacks—their disease is termed *primary progressive MS* (progression following relapses being *secondary progressive* MS). The latter presentation, substantially different from that of *relapsing-remitting MS,* presents a different set of diagnostic problems (see Chapter 4).

3.3 **Variants of demyelinating disease**

Box 3.1 Inflammatory demyelinating diseases

- Benign focal inflammatory demyelination (BFID)
  - Optic neuritis
  - Partial cord syndromes, etc
- Non-benign, non-disseminated syndromes
  - Transverse myelitis
  - Devic's disease
- Disseminated diseases
  - Acute disseminated encephalomyelitis
  - Acute haemorrhagic encephalomyelitis
  - Multiple sclerosis:
    a) Relapsing-remitting (Charcot-type) multiple sclerosis
    b) Primary progressive multiple sclerosis
    c) Marburg disease
    d) Schilder's disease
    e) (Balò's disease)

3.3.1 **Apparent variants of multiple sclerosis**

Early last century, a number of disorders were described which may be considered variants of MS. **Marburg Disease** essentially represents multiple sclerosis with a strikingly aggressive or malignant course, often rapidly fatal, often occurring after one or two isolated demyelinating events.

Schilder's diffuse sclerosis is more complex, but may represent inflammatory demyelinating disease usually of childhood onset, whose progressive course is punctuated by occasional periods of accelerated disease activity. Widespread, confluent or diffuse demyelination involving the cerebrum, cerebellum and brainstem, with pronounced axon loss and often cavitation, are characteristic features. Inherited leukodystrophies (*v.i.*) must be excluded.

Finally, **Balò's concentric sclerosis** is a pathological appearance more than a diagnosis or disease—alternating concentric rings of demyelination and apparently normal myelin—occasionally strikingly seen on MRI. Repeated inflammatory demyelinating episodes at the same site, with intervening periods of myelin repair, probably explains this architecture. No specific clinical phenotype is associated.

Retention of these terms is variable, but may be useful on clinical grounds.

3.4 **Devic's disease or neuromyelitis optica**

Eugene Devic recognized over a century ago that a group of patients with inflammatory optic nerve and spinal disease showed no evidence of disease elsewhere in the CNS. Their clinical and pathological phenotypes were clearly separable from multiple sclerosis: optic neuritis was commonly bilateral, and spinal lesions were complete rather than partial; recovery from both was often far more limited than in 'conventional' multiple sclerosis. Spinal fluid oligoclonal bands were usually absent; cranial MRI normal.

Over the last decade, circulating antibodies to an astrocyte water channel called *aquaporin-4* have been found in Devic's patients with remarkable sensitivity. Devic's disease has rapidly come to be defined by the presence of this antibody, and the phenotype has consequently evolved. Aquaporin-positive patients with either myelitis or optic neuritis alone may represent Devic's disease cases. Other clinical features have also come to be associated, including vomiting, hiccoughs, seizures, and encephalopathy; and MRI changes characteristic of Devic's rather than MS are also now defined. Secondary progression is very uncommon. The antibody association has provoked efforts to treat the disease by targeting the humoral immune system, with plasma exchange and anti-CD20 monoclonal antibodies, with some apparent success.

Other inflammatory disorders may cause a similar clinical picture, notoriously SLE, but also vasculitic syndromes, sarcoidosis, and Behçet's Disease. Usually, but not invariably, systemic or serological manifestations are apparent.

3.5 **Transverse myelitis**

'Idiopathic' transverse myelitis usually exhibits a rather different clinical phenotype to the spinal cord relapse of multiple sclerosis. In approximately 80% of cases, the thoracic cord is affected, and as the name suggests, the usual clinical picture suggests involvement of the whole transverse extent of the spinal cord. The usual picture is therefore one of rapidly progressing paralysis, sensory loss and incontinence, often with back pain, fever and sometimes meningism. Objectively, the flaccid paraparetic or paraplegic picture of spinal shock with useless bladder and/or bowel sphincters is found, with a sensory level accompanied by a band of hyperaesthesia, allodynia or hyperpathia. In multiple sclerosis, partial cord lesions are much more typical—causing a pure sensory disturbance in both legs, or deafferentation of one arm; spinal shock is quite uncommon.

A history of preceding infection (usually respiratory) in approximately one third of cases helps to emphasize the closer affinity with acute disseminated encephalomyelitis (ADEM) than multiple sclerosis, a relationship further substantiated by a more destructive histopathological picture. MR scanning too reveals a more destructive inflammatory process, far more extensive longitudinally (3 or 4 segments or more) than the clinical picture (or the name) implies. Primary causes—infections, including zoster, retroviruses, both HIV and HTLV-1, and systemic inflammatory disorders, most notoriously systemic lupus erythematosus—must be excluded. SLE can cause a severe and acute myelopathy. Spinal cord ischaemia, unless signposted by an obvious precipitant (an expanding and or dissecting aortic aneurysm, for example) can be more difficult to exclude with any certainty. Aquaporin antibody testing should nowadays be routine.

3.6 **Diffuse or disseminated syndromes**

Acute disseminated encephalomyelitis (ADEM) (Table 3.1) occurs predominantly, though by no means exclusively, in childhood—perhaps since the commonest viral precipitants of post-infectious encephalomyelitis are the childhood exanthemata. Measles virus infection is followed by ADEM in approximately 1 in 1,000 cases; the incidences of ADEM after varicella-zoster and rubella virus infections are widely quoted as 1 in 10,000 and 1 in 20,000 respectively. Other infectious (or para-infectious) precipitants include mycoplasma (and other atypical pneumonic infections), Herpesviruses, leptospira, and borrelia. ADEM also occurs as post-vaccination encephalomyelitis (perhaps 1–2 per million for live measles vaccinations). However, in a proportion of cases, no antecedent immunological challenge is identifiable. Typically, between two and 21 days after a self-limiting viral illness, there emerges a prodrome of fever, myalgia, and malaise, lasting a few days. Subsequently, acutely progressing neurological features occur whose nature indicates severe simultaneous or rapidly sequential multifocal CNS disease. Focal brainstem and/ or hemisphere signs, transverse myelitis and cranial neuropathies, including bilateral optic neuritis (unilateral disease is uncommon in this context), are seen. Cerebellar ataxia is particularly associated with varicella (and a good prognosis).

(A specific childhood ADEM phenotype was recently proposed. A small number of children were reported who developed a clinically typical ADEM presentation but with prominent additional features of a dystonic extra-pyramidal syndrome (70%) or behavioural disorder such as emotional lability or inappropriate speech (50%) in association with Group A β-haemolytic streptococcal acute pharyngitis. The syndrome was considered distinct from rheumatic fever or Sydenham's chorea, and was associated with elevated antibasal ganglia antibodies. *PANDAS syndrome*—Paediatric Autoimmune Neuropsychiatric Disorders Associated with Streptococcus infection was a suggested acronym. However there are significant questions of the existence of this as a discrete syndrome.)

Table 3.1 Comparative features of ADEM and MS

	More likely in ADEM	More likely in MS
Age	Children	Adults
Sex	Slight male preponderance in children reversed in adults	Approximately twice as common in women
Symptoms	Antecedent infection Antecedent immunisation Usually more severe Fever Headache Meningism Coma Brainstem symptoms Seizures Multifocal neurological deficit Bilateral optic neuritis	Usually less severe at onset Unilateral optic neuritis Slowly progressive symptoms

Table 3.1 (*Contd.*)		
	More likely in ADEM	**More likely in MS**
CSF	Pleocytosis Raised albumin fraction Raised protein	Oligoclonal bands

MRI	Larger lesions
	Mass effect and oedema
	Grey matter involvement
	Uniform gadolinium
	  enhancement
	Normal or resolving follow up
	  scan (no new lesions)
		Periventricular lesions
		Heterogeneous gadolinium
		  enhancement
		T1 hypointensities
		  ('black holes')
		New lesions on follow
		  up scan

Less focally, there may occur an encephalopathy (which may progress to coma), meningism, and seizures; these, the bilateral nature of optic neuritis, and the multifocal nature of the disorder (acute episodes in multiple sclerosis are usually symptomatically single-sited) all suggest ADEM rather than MS. Uncommonly, ADEM can relapse persistently, rendering the distinction from MS very difficult indeed, though so-called MDEM (multi-phasic disseminated encephalomyelitis) does probably represent a separate disorder. The spinal fluid, often cellular, usually contains no oligoclonal bands. Multifocal MRI lesions are observed, but are often more extensive and symmetrical in the white matter, and occasionally in the basal ganglia, than in multiple sclerosis. Gadolinium enhancement can also help to distinguish the disorders—a mixture of enhancing and non-enhancing lesions implies the temporal dissemination of multiple sclerosis.

Although spontaneous recovery is the rule, a fatal outcome is seen in approximately 10–20%. This may be improving, however, particularly in childhood disease—three recent studies encompassing 150 children with ADEM reported no deaths. **Corticosteroids** are widely considered to be an effective first line treatment for ADEM, and almost invariably used first line: intravenous methylprednisolone 1g daily for at least three days is advised. **Plasma exchange** is recommended in patients who respond poorly to intravenous corticosteroids.

Acute haemorrhagic leukoencephalomyelitis, or Weston-Hurst disease, is a rare, more severe (indeed commonly fatal) disorder, a hyperacute form of ADEM. The course is more rapid, with pronounced systemic features; seizures are frequent and coma usual. CSF analysis often reveals a raised intracranial pressure, and a pleomorphic cellular reaction with lymphocytes, neutrophils and significant numbers of red cells, reflecting the micro-haemorrhagic process.

3.7 Inherited disorders which may be confused with mutliple sclerosis

Adrenoleukodystrophy and *metachromatic leukodystrophy* may both cause a picture resembling multiple sclerosis. Slowly progressive disease is the rule, mimicking primary progressive MS, but remitting disease is recognized. A family history, abdominal symptoms, skin pigmentation or other Addisonian features, and absent oligoclonal bands should stimulate a search for very long chain fatty acids and/or leukocyte enzyme abnormalities. Additionally, MRI in leukodystrophies usually has at least partial specificity. Female carriers of the adrenoleukodystrophy gene can manifest. Electrophysiological evidence of a peripheral neuropathy also points to these disorders when confusion arises.

Mitochondrial disease can also cause a relapsing-remitting multifocal neurological picture. Again useful distinguishing features are described, and oligoclonal bands mostly negative. *Leber's disease* is usually readily distinguished from MS. However, an interesting variant—*Harding's disease*—has emerged in recent years. Females present with disease consistent with MS but with a particular burden on the optic nerves; CSF oligoclonal bands and cranial MRI changes suggest MS, but genetic tests reveal the presence of Leber's mitochondrial mutations.

Suggested reading

Costello D.J., Eichler A.F., Eichler F.S. (2009) Leukodystrophies: classification, diagnosis, and treatment. *Neurologist* **15**(6): 319–28.

Dale R.C., de Sousa C., Chong W.K., Cox T.C.S., Harding B., Neville B.G.R. (2000) Acute disseminated encephalomyelitis, multiphasic disseminated encephalomyelitis and multiple sclerosis in children. *Brain* **123**: 2407–22.

Ebers, G.C. (senior author) The natural history of multiple sclerosis: a geographically based study—1–10. Ten remarkable papers, all in *Brain*, over the period 1989–2010.

Frohman E.M., Wingerchuk D.M. (2010) Clinical practice. Transverse myelitis. *N Engl J Med* **363**(6): 564–72.

Hu W., Lucchinetti C.F. (2009) The pathological spectrum of CNS inflammatory demyelinating diseases. *Semin Immunopathol* **31**(4): 439–53.

Pittock S.J. (2008) Neuromyelitis optica: a new perspective. *Semin Neurol* **28**(1): 95–104.

Scolding N. (2001) The differential diagnosis of multiple sclerosis. *J Neurol Neurosurg Psychiatry* **71**(2): ii9–ii15.

Scolding N. (1999) *Immunological and Inflammatory Disorders of the Central Nervous System*. Butterworth Heinemann.

Tremlett H., Zhao Y., Rieckmann P., Hutchinson M. (2010) New perspectives in the natural history of multiple sclerosis. *Neurology* **74**(24): 2004–15.

Chapter 4

Diagnosis and differential diagnosis

> **Key points**
> - MS remains a clinical diagnosis, usually supported by investigations including MRI, LP, and evoked potentials
> - Various clinical features might raise suspicion of alternative diagnoses
> - The differential diagnosis of relapsing-remitting MS is quite different to that of primary progressive disease
> - A number of systemic inflammatory disorders can involved the central nervous system and can cause clinical pictures with significant similarities to MS
> - In many of these disorders, *presentation* with neurological problems, or disease activity confined to the nervous system, creates particular diagnostic difficulties.

31

4.1 Making the diagnosis of multiple sclerosis

The diagnosis of multiple sclerosis is often straightforward. Conventionally, it is clinically based, on the evidence of at least two demyelinating lesions presenting as distinct events affecting different areas of the CNS ('separation in time and space'). By definition, MS therefore cannot be clinically diagnosed in a patient presenting after a first solitary episode. Also, it can be difficult to know how to judge a history which is compatible with a previous event but has no contemporary objective assessment. Also, as mentioned, not all episodes of focal neurological disturbance represent inflammatory demyelination. The range of disorders which *can* mimic multiple sclerosis is enormous. Investigations are vital therefore, including MRI in virtually all suspected patients, blood tests, and often a lumbar puncture and/or clinical neurophysiological measurement of evoked potentials.

4.1.1 **MRI findings**

Patches of CNS inflammation are visible on MRI as hyper-intense T2 lesions with a characteristic distribution in the cord, corpus callosum and juxta-cortical region (Figures 4.1, 4.2). Gadolinium enhancement highlights *active* inflammation, and can be useful in identifying new lesions. Over 95% of MS patients have MRI lesions at presentation—so a normal scan does not rule out MS.

In individuals presenting with a single episode—say, optic neuritis, such multifocal white matter lesions are seen 50–70% of cases. Their presence indicates an 82% risk of developing MS in five years (i.e., having a second clinical episode), while this risk with a normal brain MRI is between 6 and 24% at five years.

There has been a trend towards diagnosing MS in some individuals according to consensus ('McDonald'; Table 4.1) criteria following a single clinical episode if subsequent MRI scanning shows the later emergence of new asymptomatic lesions. This can lead to over-diagnosis.

Fig. 4.1 a and b T2-weighted MRI scan showing white matter lesions (arrows) in a distribution typical of MS

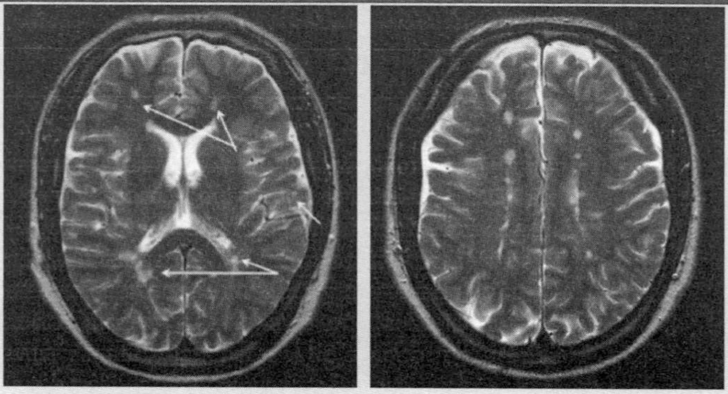

4.1.2 **CSF analysis**

Electrophoretic analysis revealing the presence of oligoclonal IgG bands in CSF that are not present in serum is seen in around 95% of MS patients. A modest number of lymphocytes (rarely above 50/mm^3) may be seen, particularly at presentation.

4.1.3 **Neurophysiological measurements**

Demyelination delays the latencies of visual, auditory and somatosensory evoked potentials, as well as central motor conduction times; wave form is well preserved.

Fig. 4.2 T2-weighted MRI scan showing a typical cervical cord plaque of multiple sclerosis (arrowed)

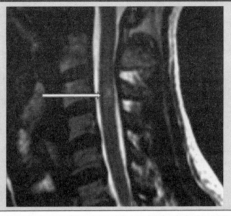

Table 4.1 The revised McDonald criteria, 2005

Clinical presentation	Additional data for MS diagnosis
Two or more attacks; objective clinical evidence of two or more lesions	None
Two or more attacks; objective clinical evidence of one lesion	Dissemination in space, demonstrated by: • MRI *or* • Two or more MRI-detected lesions consistent with MS plus positive CSF *or* • Await further clinical attack implicating a different site
One attack; objective clinical evidence of two or more lesions	Dissemination in time, demonstrated by: • MRI *or* • Second clinical attack
One attack; objective clinical evidence of one lesion (monosymptomatic presentation; clinically isolated syndrome)	Dissemination in space, demonstrated by: • MRI *or* • Two or more MRI-detected lesions consistent with MS plus positive CSF *and* Dissemination in time, demonstrated by: • MRI *or* • Second clinical attack
Insidious neurological progression suggestive of MS	One year of disease progression (retrospectively or prospectively determined) *and* Two of the following: a) Positive brain MRI (nine T2 lesions or four or more T2 lesions with positive VEP) b) Positive spinal cord MRI (two focal T2 lesions) c) Positive CSF

4.2 **The differential diagnosis of MS**

Occasionally, a very atypical (or normal) MRI scan gives rise to doubt. Additionally, an unexpected symptom or sign—fever, rash, headache, seizures, etc, or a rogue test—a raised ESR for example, can prompt the search for alternative diagnoses (see Table 4.2).

Table 4.2 Features which might lead to doubt concerning a diagnosis of multiple sclerosis*	
Systemic features	*Family history* *Fever*/night sweats, *weight loss*, arthropathy, rash, ulcers, dry mouth and eyes, ocular disease
Neurological features	*Persistent headache, seizures, encephalopathy, meningism, movement disorders*, stroke-like events, peripheral neuropathy
Investigations	Raised ESR and/or CRP, serology; abnormal CXR *Absent oligoclonal bands* or persistent CSF pleocytosis *Normal MRI or pronounced meningeal enhancement*

* (NB. Unfortunately, all of the features shown in italics can, if sometimes rarely or indirectly, as part of the response to the disease, occur in multiple sclerosis!)

Two common clinical scenarios are worth notes of their own.

First, the clinical syndrome of **optic neuritis** is not always a manifestation of idiopathic inflammatory demyelination. Identifiable primary causes include **Leber's hereditary optic neuropathy (LHON)**, typically causing bilateral simultaneous or rapidly sequential optic neuritis (unusual in multiple sclerosis, and a feature which should prompt a more intense search for primary causes), which is very severe (and usually permanent) in young men. LHON may be spotted by careful fundoscopy (preferably using a slit lamp), which shows tortuous vessels with capillary dilatation and telangiectasia, with no increase in vascular permeability apparent on fluorescein angiography, contrasting with optic neuritis. These changes are not invariable, and mitochondrial DNA analysis allows diagnostic confirmation.

Other causes include toxins (most notoriously **tobacco amblyopia** and **methanol**); **B12 deficiency**; other inflammatory disorders (particularly **sarcoidosis**, **vasculitis** and **lupus**); infections (uncommon); **ischaemia** (less uncommon, usually revealing itself by a typically vascular more abrupt onset, an absence of pain, and a horizontal altitudinal field defect; and optic nerve, chiasmal or other local **tumours**. These may be intrinsic (classically **gliomata** or **optic nerve sheath meningiomata**, the latter suggested by the presence of opto-ciliary shunt vessels) or extrinsic (**pituitary tumours** and **craniopharyngiomata**).

Secondly, diagnosing **primary progressive multiple sclerosis** presents a different set of problems. The clinical picture is not especially characteristic, and alternative diagnoses are therefore generally sought more actively. Most patients with a progressive paraparesis would routinely undergo spinal cord MR imaging, which will exclude many (surgically relevant) causes; adding brain examination will help confirm the diagnosis. Both cerebral and spinal appearances of B12 deficiency can resemble those of MS (and the ankle jerks are not always absent in early deficiency, though glossitis usually is), so that checking B12 levels is mandatory. HTLV-related myelopathy can likewise cause similar brain and spine MR changes, and in this instance CSF oligoclonal bands are present: HTLV serology is therefore also recommended. Other systemic inflammatory diseases should be actively sought. Hereditary diseases are not always conveniently flagged by a family history, absent ankle jerks and pes cavus, but cerebral MRI and the presence of oligoclonal bands usually make the distinction straightforward. (Note that the VER can be abnormal in some of the spinocerebellar ataxias.) Genetic testing for these (including various spinocerebellar ataxias) is available.

4.3 **Disorders which may mimic MS**

4.3.1 **Other inflammatory disorders**

4.3.1.1 Cerebral vasculitis

Vasculitis is neither a diagnosis or disease, but a histopathological process (Table 4.3). In both isolated CNS vasculitis and CNS involvement in systemic vasculitis, three broad clinical phenotypes are proposed. Tumour-like lesions, and acute encephalopathies rarely suggest MS, but the third is often mistaken. The 'MS-plus' presentation of CNS vasculitis includes a relapsing-remitting course, and features such as optic neuropathy and brain stem episodes. However, additional features less common in MS also occur—seizures, severe, persisting headaches (80% or more patients), encephalopathic episodes, or hemispheric stroke-like events. Systemic features may also be present (often revealed only on direct enquiry) even in so-called isolated CNS vasculitis—fever and night sweats, skin or eye changes, oligoarthropathy—also contrasting with MS.

Table 4.3 Classification of vasculitis

Dominant vessel involved	Primary	Secondary
Large arteries	Giant cell arteritis Takayasu's arteritis	Aortitis with rheumatoid disease; infection (e.g. syphilis)
Medium arteries	Classical polyarteritis nodosa Kawasaki disease	Infection (e.g. Hepatitis B)
Small vessels and medium arteries	Wegener's granulomatosis Churg-Strauss syndrome Microscopic polyangiitis **Idiopathic CNS angiitis**	Vasculitis in rheumatoid disease, SLE, Sjögren's syndrome, drugs, infection (e.g. HIV)
Small vessels	Henoch-Schönlein purpura Essential cryoglobulinaemia Cutaneous leukocytoclastic vasculitis	Drugs (e.g. sulphonamides, etc.) Infection (e.g. Hepatitis C)

The diagnosis of isolated/primary cerebral vasculitis can be very difficult (systemic vasculitis 'spilling over' into the CNS is usually more straightforward). Serological markers, including ANCA are commonly negative. Spinal fluid examination is, like ESR, usually abnormal, but lacks specificity, along with changes in cell count, protein and/or immunoglobulin band analysis. MRI can closely resemble MS—but may be normal. Contrast angiography often shows segmental (often multifocal) narrowing and areas of localised dilatation or beading, and occlusion, rarely also with aneurysms. Whilst these changes are also non-specific, they are not seen in multiple sclerosis. However, the false negative rate for angiography is at least 30%. Histopathological confirmation, biopsying a lesion where possible, otherwise by 'blind' biopsy incorporating meninges, and non-dominant temporal white and grey matter, therefore can be important, though not a trivial or frontal procedure. The distinction is, of course, important. Cyclophosphamide (with corticosteroids) is of value in confirmed vasculitis.

4.3.1.2 Systemic lupus erythematosus (SLE)

The term *lupoid sclerosis*—MS-like neurological features in the context of known SLE—is neither accurate nor useful. Primary demyelination is not seen in CNS-lupus; low level positive ANA serological tests are common and do not prove SLE. MS and SLE are separate diseases. Neurological involvement in SLE is common, but neurological presentation much less so—as with vasculitis, neurological disease in the setting of known lupus presents less of a problem. It is uncommon therefore for lupus and MS to be confused diagnostically.

Box 4.1 Lupoid sclerosis

The term *lupoid sclerosis*—MS-like neurological features in the context of known SLE—is neither accurate nor useful. Primary demyelination is not seen in CNS-lupus; low level positive ANA serological tests are common and do not prove SLE. MS and SLE are separate diseases.

Direct enquiry and focussed systemic examination should disclose fever, malaise, skin changes (classically, the malar butterfly rash and/or photosensitivity) and arthritis. Revised SLE diagnostic criteria, with an estimated specificity and sensitivity of 96%, are widely accepted (see American College of Rheumatology diagnostic criteria for SLE). Importantly, most authorities suggest that only ANA titres over 1:160 are diagnostically relevant.

Box 4.2 American College of Rheumatology diagnostic criteria for SLE

'a person shall be said to have SLE if four or more of the 11 criteria are present, serially or simultaneously, during any interval of observation'
- malar flush
- discoid rash
- photosensitivity
- oral ulcers
- arthritis
- serositis (pleurisy or pericarditis)
- renal disorder (proteinuria >0.5g/24h or cellular casts)
- neurological disorder (seizures, psychosis; *other causes excluded;* [author's italics])
- haematological disorder (haemolytic anaemia, leucopoenia or lymphopoenia on two or more occasions, or thrombocytopoenia)
- immunological disorder—LE cells, or anti-dsDNA or anti-Sm or persistent false positive syphilis serology
- anti-nuclear autoantibodies.

Ataxia, brain stem syndromes, and cranial neuropathies may resemble MS, but more particularly associated with lupus are *optic neuropathy* and *transverse myelopathy*. The former is often painless (unlike MS), sub-acute and progressive, and commonly very severe; the latter usually resembles idiopathic transverse myelitis more than spinal relapses of MS. Headache, seizures, psychiatric and cognitive disturbances are relatively common in SLE but not MS, as are episodes of encephalopathy, and movement disorders (especially chorea). Stroke, particularly in antiphospholipid syndrome, rarely of course resembles MS.

A persistently raised ESR and serological changes are seen (Table 4.4), and CSF protein level may be raised, with a neutrophil or lymphocyte pleocytosis. Oligoclonal band analysis is positive in up to 50% patients with CNS lupus. Interestingly and unlike MS, these changes can resolve with successful immunotherapy. (The same applies to sarcoidosis and vasculitis.) MRI changes are neither invariable nor specific. Skin biopsy (staining for complement deposition) can be extremely helpful in suspected but elusive lupus.

CNS involvement in lupus almost always reflects microvascular thrombotic damage, not vasculitis. It is a poor prognostic sign in SLE.

Table 4.4 **Autoantibodies and their connective tissue disease associations**

Immunofluorescence pattern	Antibody	Disease associations
Rim ANA	anti-native DNA (anti-dsDNA)	SLE (50%)
Homogeneous ANA	anti-histone	Drug-induced lupus (97%) **N.B. low titre (<1:320) in normals**
speckled ANA	anti-Ro (SS-A)	Sjögren's (75%) SLE (30%)
	anti-La (SS-B)	Sjögren's (60%) SLE (15%)
	anti-Scl-70	systemic sclerosis (50%)
	anti-Sm	SLE (75%)
	anti-RNP (anti-U1-nRNP)	MCTD (95%) SLE (30%)
Nucleolar ANA	anti-PM-Scl	?identifies polymyositis/ scleroderma overlap
Other organelles	anti-centromere	systemic sclerosis (85%)

4.3.1.3 Sjögren's syndrome

Sjögren's syndrome comprises keratoconjunctivitis sicca, and xerostomia occurring (in some 50% of cases) with another connective tissue disorder, usually rheumatoid arthritis. Speckled anti-Ro (SS-A) or anti-La (SS-B) antibodies are present. Any neurological manifestations are usually peripheral; trigeminal neuropathy is classically described. An MS-like picture has been reported (optic neuropathy is particularly associated), but symptoms of dry mouth and eyes, and the serological changes, mean that persistent diagnostic confusion is not common.

4.3.1.4 Neurosarcoidosis

Sarcoidosis affects the nervous system in approximately 5% of patients. Optic nerve disease is particularly associated; a chronic progressive course, and persistent steroid sensitivity commonly point away from MS. Cognitive and neuropsychiatric abnormalities, and peripheral involvement (nerve and muscle) are also unlike MS. However, other cranial neuropathies (especially the facial nerve), and brain stem and spinal cord disease may variably resemble MS.

The chest x-ray is abnormal in less than 50% of patients, but CT is more sensitive (subclinical thoracic disease is said to be present in most cases of extrathoracic sarcoidosis). Searching for anterior and/or posterior segment inflammation using slit lamp examination and fluorescein angiography can be valuable. Serum and CSF angiotensin coverting enzyme (ACE) levels may be elevated; the CSF may reveal increases in protein or cell count in 80% of cases. Oligoclonal bands may be present, though as with other non-MS pathologies, their presence varies when serially assessed. Whole body gallium scanning can disclose asymptomatic foci of systemic disease. Cranial MRI may show multiple white matter lesions and/or, in about a third of patients, meningeal enhancement (Figure 4.3). The diagnosis is confirmed where possible by biopsy, either of cerebral or meningeal tissue, or of lung or conjunctiva where appropriate.

4.3.1.5 Behçet's disease

Behçet's disease is a chronic relapsing multisystem inflammatory disorder. Some 5% of patients develop neurological complications, include cerebral venous sinus thrombosis, sterile meningoencephalitis, encephalopathy, and psychiatric and progressive cognitive manifestations. MRI abnormalities are non-specific, though posterior fossa and brainstem involvement is said to be typical. Oligoclonal bands are uncommon.

4.3.1.6 Whipple's disease

Whipple's disease, caused by Tropheryma whippelii, causes arthropathy, respiratory symptoms, anaemia, fever, erythema nodosum, and severe wasting, in addition to steatorrhoea and abdominal distension. 10% of patients have neurological involvement; 5% present in this way. A wide variety of features is seen; but few resemble MS.

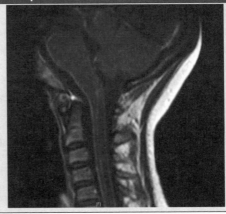

Fig. 4.3 Extensive leptomeningeal enhancement over the surface of the spinal cord and brain stem in neurosarcoidosis

---

Box 4.3 Behçet's disease diagnostic criteria

- Recurrent oral ulceration (at least three times in one year) is an absolute criterion;
- Plus any two of:
  - Recurrent genital ulceration
  - Uveitis or retinal vasculitis
- Skin lesions
  - [erythema nodosum
  - acneiform nodules
  - pseudofolliculitis or
  - papulopustular lesions]
- A positive pathergy test (read at 24–48 hours)

CSF samples may reveal pathognomic PAS-positive bacilli; small bowel or lymph node biopsy (with electron microscopy) can be diagnostic. Polymerase chain reaction analysis of blood, lymph node, spinal fluid, small bowel tissue or brain is increasingly used.

4.3.2 **Vascular disease**

Arteriovenous malformations enjoyed a certain notoriety as a confounding cause of a relapsing remitting single-sited syndrome but much less so post-MRI. *SBE* and *atrial myxoma* can rarely cause a more challenging picture through multifocal embolic infarction. *CADASIL* can mislead, but the family history, cognitive features, usually distinctive MRI changes, and absence of oligoclonal bands should arouse suspicion.

> **Box 4.4 Neurological features of Whipple's disease (in approximate order of frequency)**
>
> Cognitive changes, dementia and/or psychiatric disease
> Supranuclear gaze palsy
> Pyramidal signs
> Hypothalamic features
> — somnolence, polydipsia, increased appetite, hypogonadism
> Myoclonus
> Oculo-masticatory myorhythmia
> Cranial neuropathies.
> Seizures
> Eye disease
> — keratitis, uveitis, papilloedema, ptosis
> Ataxia

4.3.2.1 Foix-Alajuanine syndrome

Foix and Alajouanine described *sub-acute necrotic myelitis*. This predominantly affects adult males, with spastic paralysis, sensory loss, and incontinence progressing over two to three months; a flaccid, areflexic, amyotrophic phase ensue. Systemic features—fever, meningism and often severe local pain, are common. Spinal fluid changes (markedly elevated protein levels but few or normal cells)—and in later cases, imaging—reflect spinal block from a markedly swollen cord. Neuropathologically, there is a severe necrotic process affecting grey and white matter, putatively reflecting a veno-occlusive cause: thrombin deposition, with thickening the walls of vessels, is often prominent.

4.3.3 Infectious diseases

While the commoner acute presentation of meningism (or meningoencephalitis), facial palsy and/or painful radiculopathy presents few problems, so-called tertiary *Lyme disease*, with progressive syndromes including spastic paraparesis, cerebellar ataxia and recurrent cranial neuropathies, can cause diagnostic confusion. MRI can show multifocal white matter lesions, and the CSF can contain oligoclonal bands. The cell count is often persistently high, however. A history of the characteristic skin rash several years earlier will not be mentioned unless directly queried. Serological tests on both blood and CSF are therefore important; PCR also plays a role. *Neurosyphilis* is increasing in frequency though still earns mention mostly through historic respect, rarely causing a picture easily confused with MS, particularly in the MRI era. Headache and seizures are common, and pupillary abnormalities are, of course, characteristic. Syphilitic optic neuritis is usually painless.

4.3.4 **Malignancy**

A number of CNS malignancies carry reputations as mimics of MS, but most of these have failed to survive the widespread availability of MRI. *Meningiomata* can cause relapsing (unifocal) disease—most notoriously in pregnancy, as a presumed consequence of the oestrogen receptors they express. *Gliomata*, especially in the brainstem, can also show this course. *Epidermoid cysts of the IVth ventricle* may trap the unwary, and most neurologists have a healthy respect for *foramen magnum tumours*. *Chiari malformations* include Lhermitte's sign and trigeminal neuralgia among symptoms of particular relevance in the current context. None, however, easily evade the MR scanner. One of the few primary CNS malignancies that can is the *multifocal glioma*.

Paraneoplastic leukocytoclastic vasculitis (which is rarely neurological) may complicate a variety of cancers, and CNS angiitis associated with *Hodgkin's disease* is reported. *Lymphomatoid granulomatosis* is a rare T-lymphoma centred on the vascular wall, while *neoplastic or malignant angioendotheliosis,* also rare, is a B-cell lymphoma, where the neoplastic process is intraluminal. As with other CNS vasculopathies, all *can* cause a picture resembling MS. Systemic features—low grade or undulating fever, weight loss, pruritis—should raise suspicions. Other paraneoplastic disorders rarely permit serious confusion with MS, though cancer-related retinopathy can superficially resemble optic neuritis.

4.4 **Disclosing a diagnosis of MS**

In reality, having excluded other disorders as mentioned, one is commonly left with two options: MS or *possible* MS. Whether and or when to declare the latter is difficult: most would rather not offer the diagnosis of an incurable and often disabling disease unless absolutely certain. But one large study has shown that the majority of MS patients (91%) would prefer to be given the diagnosis as soon as it is even suspected—though it was conducted in patients who ultimately did have a diagnosis of MS. NICE guidelines also recommend that patients should be informed of the possibility of MS. Familiarity with the natural history and prognosis of MS can help to reassure the patient. Further support for the patient, their families and friends, can be obtained from specialist MS nurses, the established societies and their websites.

Suggested reading

Akman-Demir G., Serdaroglu P., Tasçi B. (1999) Clinical patterns of neurological involvement in Behçet's disease: evaluation of 200 patients. The Neuro-Behçet Study Group. *Brain* **122**: 2171–82.

Awad A., Hemmer B., Hartung H.P., Kieseier B., Bennett J.L., Stuve O. (2010) Analyses of cerebrospinal fluid in the diagnosis and monitoring of multiple sclerosis. *J Neuroimmunol* **219**(1–2): 1–7.

Joseph F.G., Scolding N.J. (2010) *Neurolupus Pract Neurol* **10**(1): 4–15.

Joseph F.G., Scolding N.J. (2007) Sarcoidosis of the nervous system. *Pract Neurol* **7**(4): 234–44.

Leocani L., Comi G. (2000) Neurophysiological investigations in multiple sclerosis. *Curr Opin Neurol* **13**(3): 255–61.

Miller D.H., Leary S.M. (2007) Primary-progressive multiple sclerosis. *Lancet Neurol* **6**(10): 903–12.

Panegyres P.K., Edis R., Beaman M., Fallon M. (2006) Primary Whipple's disease of the brain: characterization of the clinical syndrome and molecular diagnosis. *QJM* **99**(9): 609–23.

Papathanasopoulos P.G., Nikolakopoulou A., Scolding N.J. (2005) Disclosing the diagnosis of multiple sclerosis. *J Neurol* **252**(11): 1307–9.

Scoldng N. (2001) The differential diagnosis of multiple sclerosis. *J Neurol Neurosurg Psychiatry* **71**(2): ii9–ii15.

Scolding N.J. (2009) Central nervous system vasculitis. *Semin Immunopathol* **31**(4): 527–36.

Traboulsee A.L., Li D.K. (2006) The role of MRI in the diagnosis of multiple sclerosis. *Adv Neurol* **98**: 125–46.

Chapter 5

Treating multiple sclerosis

> **Key points**
> - MS therapies either treat the effects of the disease (symptomatic treatments) or modulate disease processes (disease-modifying therapies)
> - Symptomatic therapies often involve a multi-disciplinary approach
> - Currently licensed disease-modifying therapies reduce relapse rates in MS
> - The effects of current disease-modifying therapies on long-term disability are yet to be fully understood.

The treatment of multiple sclerosis currently falls into two categories: treating the effects of neurological damage caused by the disease (symptomatic therapies); and modulating the disease process (disease-modifying therapies). In recent years significant advances have been made in developing therapeutic strategies for the latter. Only 18 years ago, a patient diagnosed with multiple sclerosis could be offered little in the way of treatment which could alter the natural history of the disease. Now a number of therapies have been licensed which have varying degrees of success in modifying disease processes and many more are currently in trial stages. Despite these major advances in therapies the disease currently has no cure.

5.1 Symptomatic therapies

Patients with multiple sclerosis experience acute episodes of neurological dysfunction (relapses) and persistent symptoms. These persistent symptoms are common in the progressive phases of the disease and reflect previous or active damage to regions of the central nervous system. Common symptoms include spasticity, pain, urinary dysfunction, ataxia, fatigue, visual disturbance, paraesthesiae, sexual dysfunction, and mood disturbances. Approaches to treatment of these symptoms will often involve a range of pharmacological and non-pharmacological agents and is often best approached in a multi-disciplinary setting.

5.1.1 Spasticity

Spasticity arises from hyper-excitability of stretch reflexes resulting in velocity-dependent increase in tone and exaggerated reflexes. It is found in a variety of 'upper motor neuron' syndromes and is thought to be mainly generated via loss of descending inhibition on reflex arcs. In MS the clinical phenotypes of spastic paraparesis or quadriparesis are common and predominantly reflect spinal cord disease. Spasticity in association with hemiparesis or even single limb spasticty is also seen. As with many symptomatic therapies in multiple sclerosis, a multi-disciplinary approach to spasticity is optimal and physiotherapists play an important role. Prior to commencement of therapy, an assessment and agreement on the desired functional impact of the therapy should be discussed. For instance, for some patients a major goal may be to improve seating posture, whilst for others it may be to reduce painful spasms.

5.1.1.1 Therapies for spasticity
Physical therapies

Physiotherapy and exercise are important methods of managing muscle stiffness and are often used in combination with pharmacological therapies. Because of the broad range of symptoms and disabilities in MS, individually tailored physiotherapy programmes with specific goals are set following a comprehensive assessment of functional disturbances. Types of exercises used in physiotherapy include passive and active stretching, muscle strengthening, postural exercises, aerobic activities (e.g. cycling) and 'range-of-motion' exercises during which joints are made to go through full ranges of movements. Randomized control trials of physiotherapy in MS have been performed which have backed up the view that a variety of physiotherapy techniques are helpful for persistent symptoms and may specifically help quality of life scores, gait and spasticity. Secondary effects such as reduction in osteoporosis and improvements in cardiovascular health by increasing ambulation may also be seen. Some studies have reported that physiotherapy in addition to steroid therapy during acute relapses may help. Many patients with MS experience Uhthoff's phenomenon (increase in symptoms associated with an elevated body core temperature) which may limit exercise.

5.1.1.2 Drug therapies
Baclofen

- *Oral*: baclofen is a GABA$_B$ agonist which is thought to act by decreasing neuronal excitability in the dorsal horn of the spinal cord.

It is the most commonly used first-line drug for generalized spasticity. Typically the dose is titrated slowly until reaching maximal effect. The major limitation of the use of baclofen, as with most anti-spasm medications, is the induction of muscle weakness and most patients will not tolerate doses above 80–90 mg per 24 hours. Reduction in muscle tone reduces some of the 'splinting' effects that spasticity has on the legs and reducing spasticity may paradoxically increase disability. Baclofen may also reduce truncal tone, which may impair sitting. Other side effects include: dizziness, drowsiness, urinary frequency, and headache. Rarely, baclofen may induce seizures

- *Intrathecal*: delivery of baclofen directly into the spinal fluid is an option for patients with severe spasticity. Intrathecal baclofen (ITB) has the advantage of allowing very low doses to be used with minimal systemic side effects. ITB is delivered using a pump which is implanted intra-abdominally and a catheter which passes into the spinal cerebrospinal fluid. The rates of administration can be varied and the pump has to be refilled periodically. Prior to insertion of an ITB, rigorous assessments of spasticity must be made and test doses of ITB are carried out with physician assessment. Although usually well tolerated, side effects such as nausea, drowsiness, urinary retention, and hypotension are sometimes reported. In rare cases of pump malfunction, the potentially serious problem of baclofen withdrawal, characterized by rebound spasticity, confusion, seizures, and rarely multi-organ failure, may occur. Expense is a significant factor.

Tizanidine

Tizanidine is an α_2-adrenergic receptor agonist which has a similar clinical efficacy to baclofen but is often better tolerated. It is thought that tizanidine increases inhibition of spinal noradrenergic neurons with a net reduction in the facilitation of spinal motor neurons. Trials of tizanidine have demonstrated equal efficacy of the drug when compared to baclofen, accompanied by a decrease in adverse events leading to trial withdrawal. Tizanidine usage is generally accompanied by less motor weakness than that seen with baclofen. Side effects include somnolence, dizziness, and dry mouth. Approximately 5% of patients treated with tizanidine experience elevation in liver enzymes which typically reverses on withdrawal of the drug. As a result liver function should be monitored regularly in those receiving the drug.

Gabapentin

Gabapentin is generally used as a second-line drug and can be particularly useful for painful spasms and if central neuropathic pain co-exists.

Dantrolene

Dantrolene acts directly on skeletal muscle and may thus avoid some of the CNS effects seen with other anti-spasticity agents. Its use is, however, associated with gastrointestinal side-effects, hepatotoxicity and, more rarely, cardio-pulmonary disease. It is now less commonly used to treat spasticity in MS, but can be useful in cases of poor tolerance to other drugs.

Benzodiazepines

Diazepam is the most commonly used benzodiazepine to treat spasticity in MS. Doses of diazepam used in spasticity are generally similar to those used in anxiety treatments. Sedation and muscle weakness are common accompaniments of diazepam use and careful and slow dose titration is needed. Clonazepam may also have a role in some patients.

Cannabinoids

Recently cannabinoids have been licensed in several countries for the management of spasticity. Sativex® (consisting of delta-9-tetra-hydrocannabinol (THC) and cannabidiol (CBD)) is an oromucosal spray which may be used as an add-on treatment for symptom improvement in MS patients with moderate to severe spasticity who have not responded adequately to other anti-spasticity medication. Several placebo-controlled trials have been performed suggesting improvements in visual analogue scales of symptoms and other spasticity rating scales. However, current evidence suggests its effects may be limited in many patients and few would recommend it as first-line therapy. Common side effects include dizziness and fatigue.

5.1.1.3 Other therapies

Botulinum toxin

Botulinum toxin blocks presynaptic release of acetylcholine at the neuromuscular junction rendering muscles weak. Two serotypes of toxin (A and B) are in clinical use and the effects of botulinum toxin usually last for approximately three months. Botulinum toxin therapy for MS is used to treat focal spasticity and may be particularly useful for leg adductor spasticity, spastic pes equinus, 'striatal' toe or adductor spasticity of the shoulder. It also has a role on occasion in managing pain caused by spasticity and, in bedridden patients, can sometimes reduce the formation of decubitus ulcers. As with all anti-spasticity agents, the efficacy of botulinum toxin is optimized by concomitant physiotherapy.

Surgical procedures

Surgical procedures, such as rhizotomy, are occasionally used to treat resistant cases of spasticity, although the evidence base for such therapies in MS is lacking.

5.1.2 Pain

Pain is a common symptom in MS and has been estimated to occur chronically in up to two-thirds of patients. Pain may occur acutely or, more commonly, in patients with chronic disease, and a number of pain syndromes occur MS. The commonest description of pain in MS is of a neuropathic quality and so-called central neuropathic pain is thought to be amongst the commonest of chronic pain mechanisms. Pain syndromes such as central dysaesthetic pain, trigeminal neuralgia, painful tonic spasms, and paroxysmal sensory disturbances such as Lhermitte's phenomenon occur in MS and have specific management issues.

5.1.2.1 Central Neuropathic Pain (CNP)

Neuropathic pain syndromes are chronic pain disorders caused as a consequence of dysfunction of parts of the nervous system that normally signal pain. With regards to MS, lesions within the spinal cord, thalamus and brainstem are thought to be more associated with pain syndromes than those elsewhere. Pain is commoner in progressive MS, particularly PPMS, and experienced to a lesser degree by those with RRMS. Most commonly patients with MS complain of dysaesthesia, typically constant burning-type pains experienced in the lower limbs, distally more than proximally. The mechanisms of central neuropathic pain in MS, however, are not fully understood although alterations in spinal and descending supraspinal modulation of pain arising as a result of inflammation and post-inflammatory scarring are likely to be important pain generators.

Table 5.1 Drugs used for the treatment of central neuropathic pain in MS

Type of drug	Drug examples	Common side effects
Tricyclic anti-depressants	Amitriptyline Nortriptyline Imipramine	dry mouth, constipation, confusion urinary retention; rarely: arhythmias
Selective noradrenaline reuptake inhibitors	Duloxetine Venlafaxine	headaches, nausea, insomnia sexual dysfunction, dry mouth
Anti-convulsants	Gabapentin Carbamazepine Pregabalin Lamotrigine Levetiracetam	Dizziness, drowsiness Unsteadiness, dizziness, drowsiness Dizziness, drowsiness Rash (seek medical advice), myalgia, headaches Paraesthesiae, anxiety

The treatment of central neuropathic pain is similar to treatment of neuropathic pain generated as a result of peripheral nerve disease. Randomized control trials of pain medications in MS are limited and treatment is often empirical. Commonly used drugs include tricyclic antidepressants and anti-epileptic medications (Table 5.1). Long-term use of analgesics including non-steroidal anti-inflammatory agents and opioids should generally be avoided due to long-term side effects and issues of tolerance. In resistant cases patients should be referred to pain clinics for rationalization of medications and consideration of non-pharmacological approaches to pain.

The use of cannibinoids for central neuropathic pain has been recently investigated and although effects are often seen, these drugs are often limited by side effects. Further studies are on-going.

5.1.2.2 *Other pain syndromes experienced in MS and treatments*

- *Trigeminal neuralgia (TN)*: although classically associated with MS, TN is not common in the disease. Treatment of TN in MS follow the same algorithm as treatment of idiopathic TN and commonly used drugs include carbamazepine, gabapentin, lamotrigine, and topiramate. Neurosurgical intervention in refractive cases can be valuable

- *Painful tonic spasms*: these are cramping, pulling pains commoner in the legs which are often stimulus sensitive. They are closely linked to spasticity. Carbamazepine is commonly used. In addition gabapentin or anti-spasticity medication (e.g. baclofen or benzodiazepines) may help

- *Optic neuritis*: the pain of optic neuritis is short lived but may respond to corticosteroids or non-steroidal anti-inflammatory drugs

- *Paroxysmal sensory disturbances*: transient sensory disturbances such as Lhermitte's phenomenon usually do not require treatment and often remit spontaneously.

5.1.3 **Urinary dysfunction**

Urinary dysfunction is amongst the commonest of symptoms experienced by patients with MS and should be asked for specifically during consultations. Common symptoms include urgency, frequency, hesitancy, incontinence, and nocturia. Urinary dysfunction occurs for a variety of reasons but is very commonly associated with spinal cord pathology and in most cases is probably due to disconnection between the brainstem micturition centres and the sacral spinal cord. Approaches to management need to be guided by the patient's overall level of disability, since treatment of very immobile patients will differ from those in the ambulant. A further consideration is that worsening of bladder function can occur due to urinary tract infections which should always be suspected. Patients with chronic urinary dysfunction as a result of MS have an increased susceptibility to urine infection. Urinary tract infection may also cause exacerbations of neurological symptoms in MS and may mimic MS relapse.

5.1.3.1 Investigations for bladder dysfunction

The therapeutic approach to management of bladder symptoms is strongly guided by simple investigations which can generally be carried out in clinic (see Figure 5.1). Central to management strategy is determining whether the patient has incomplete bladder voiding or an overactive bladder (detrusor muscle overactivity). The history of urinary dysfunction can often give clues as to the nature of the bladder problems although symptoms are often similar and assessment of post-voiding residual volume (PVR) should be carried out during initial assessments. PVR is most commonly measured by ultrasound methods and many MS specialist nurses or continence advisors are able to carry out this assessment. For more complicated urinary dysfunction or those refractory to initial therapies, urodynamic studies may be required. If the PVR is measured to be below 100 ml, the diagnosis of urinary dysfunction is more likely to be one of bladder overactivity and drug therapies, such as anti-muscarinics, are often prescribed. Conversely, a large PVR (>100 ml) suggests incomplete bladder voiding and physical methods to empty the bladder are warranted. In all patients with MS, particularly those with acute or acutely worsening urinary dysfunction, urine dipstick and/ or mid-stream urinalysis (MSU) should be performed to exclude urinary tract infections. Patients with recurrent urinary tract infections should be investigated with ultrasound and cystoscopy to check for any underlying structural abnormality. Although prophylactic antibiotics are not recommended for routine use in bladder dysfunction in MS, some patients with recurrent infection may benefit from this approach. Due to the complex nature of bladder dysfunction that occurs in MS, some patients use a combination of treatments.

5.1.3.2 Management of incomplete bladder voiding

- *Clean intermittent self-catheterization (ISC)*: if significant PVRs are measured by ultrasound ISC should be discussed. In many cases, patients themselves can be taught how to perform this technique. Sometimes a partner or other carer may perform ISC. ISC should be taught by a specialist MS or urology nurse and may be carried out several times per day. The importance of hygiene and cleanliness during ISC should be emphasized to reduce infections.

- *Long-term catheterization*: In patients whose level of disability precludes ISC long-term catheterisation may be necessary. Suprapubic insertion of the urinary catheter is generally recommended to prevent progressive urethral damage.

5.1.3.3 Management of overactive bladder

- *Anti-muscarinics*: several anti-muscarinic agents are now in clinical practice for the treatment of detrusor muscle overactivity (see Table 5.2). Anti-muscarinics block muscarinic acetylcholine receptors within bladder smooth muscle to reduce detrusor contractions and may increase bladder capacity. Both non-selective anti-muscarinics and selective M_2 and/or M_3 muscarinic antagonists are in clinic use and modified release formulations of some drugs exist. Anti-muscarinics should be used with caution in the elderly, patients with cognitive impairment and those with susceptibility to angle-closure glaucoma. In addition anti-muscarinics may worsen cardiac diseases (e.g. arrhythmias, heart failure and coronary artery disease), hypertension and hyperthyroidism. The use of anti-muscarinics is often limited by side effects which commonly include dry mouth, gastro-intestinal upset, blurred vision, drowsiness, fatigue, and dizziness.

Table 5.2 Anti-muscarinic drugs used in the management of detrusor overactivity

Drug	Trade name	Typical dose	Available as modified release formulation	Receptor sub-type antagonism
Oxybutynin hydrochloride	Ditropan®	5 mg bd/tds	Yes	Non-selective
Tolterodine tartrate	Detrusitol®	2 mg bd	Yes	Non-selective
Solifenacin succinate	Vesicare®	5–10 mg od	No (long half-life)	M_2 and M_3 selective
Darifenacin	Emselex®	7.5 mg od	No	M_3 selective
Trospium chloride	Regurin®	20 mg bd	No	Non-selective
Propiverine hydrochloride	Detrunorm®	15 mg od-tds	No	Non-selective
Fesoterodine fumarate	Toviaz®	4 mg od	No	Non-selective

5.1.3.4 Other therapies

- *Botulinum toxin injection into the detrusor muscle*: there is increasing evidence that injection of botulinum toxin A into the detrusor muscle is highly effective for severe detrusor overactivity. However the treatment remains unlicensed and only available in certain specialist centres.

- *Desmopressin*: This analogue of vasopressin (anti-diuretic hormone) has been used in some patients with MS to treat daytime frequency or nocturia. Care is needed to avoid fluid overload.
- *Physical methods*: physical interventions, such as pelvic floor exercises and 'bladder training' may have inhibitory effects on detrusor activity.

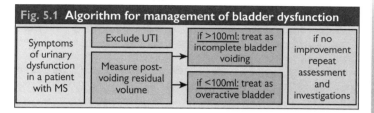

Fig. 5.1 **Algorithm for management of bladder dysfunction**

5.1.4 **Tremor and ataxia**

Tremor is a relatively common symptom in MS, particularly in those with progressive disease. Action tremors, both postural and intention, predominate since the anatomical substrate for most MS-related tremors is the cerebellum and its connections. Resting tremors are rare. Holmes' ('rubral') tremor can also occur with midbrain lesions.

The management of tremor can be difficult and in severe cases, surgical treatment may be considered. Pharmacological agents including propranolol, ondansetron, clonazepam, carbamazepine, and isoniazid have been trialled with limited proven beneficial effects. Recent trials of cannabinoids have been disappointing. Surgical treatments using thalamic stimulation (deep brain stimulation) may prove highly effective in very selective cases.

Action tremors form part of the wider symptomatology of ataxia. Associated symptoms of incoordination, dysmetria, and dysarthria are very difficult to treat and no therapy has been shown to impact significantly on these symptoms in trials. To some extent this may reflect the difficulty in conducting such trials. Physiotherapy is often used for management of ataxic symptoms and speech therapy may be useful for the management of dysarthria.

5.1.5 **Mood and cognition**

Major depression has an approximate lifetime incidence of 50% in MS. Prompt recognition and treatment of depressive symptoms is important since it is a predictor of morbidity, quality of life, drug therapy compliance and suicide risk. Psychosocial factors play a major role in the aetiology of depression in MS, as they do in most chronic diseases. Treatment of major depression follows similar lines to non-MS related depression. The most commonly used drugs are the selective serotonin reuptake inhibitors (SSRIs). A combination of anti-depressant drug therapy and some form of psychotherapy, for instance cognitive-behavioural therapy (CBT), often proves most effective.

In a similar way, impairment of cognitive function in MS has major implications on quality of life. In progressive MS, deficits in frontal executive function are most common, whereas patients with RRMS sometimes show problems with memory functions. In this latter group, however, a careful assessment for features of major depression should be carried out. Currently approved drugs for the treatment of Alzheimer's disease (acetylcholinesterase inhibitors) have been investigated in several small studies, but, at present, there is insufficient evidence to recommend their use. In a similar way, some trials have assessed the influence of beta-interferons and glatiramer acetate on cognition, and although some improvements in selected cognitive domains occurred the effect of these drugs on long-term cognitive function in MS is unclear.

5.1.6 **Fatigue and sleep disturbance**

Fatigue refers to a subjective lack of physical or mental 'energy' that impacts significantly on the ability to carry out activities of daily living. Amongst the commonest of symptoms in MS patients, and often ranked amongst the most severe in patient surveys, it can be one of the most difficult to treat. Although highly complex in its aetiology, axonal conduction block occurring in the context of demyelination may contribute to fatigue. This may help to explain why fatigue is often exacerbated by heat, activity, or relapse. Drug therapies include amantadine (mechanism unknown) and modafinil (CNS stimulant blocking noradrenaline reuptake in the hypothalamus). 4-aminopyridine and 3, 4-diaminopyridine are potassium channel blockers which improve conduction in demyelinated axons and have been trialled in MS. Although limited by side effects (paraesthesiae, hepatotoxicity, and seizures) these drugs do show some clinical effects which are accompanied by neurophysiological indicators of improved axonal conduction. Fampridine (4-aminopyridine) has recently been approved in some countries for treatment of walking disability. In all patients with fatigue investigations looking for other potentially treatable conditions, such as anaemia or thyroid disease, should be carried out.

Linking closely to daytime fatigue, sleep problems are estimated to be commoner in MS patients than in the general population, with the commonest complaint being one of insomnia. Sleep disturbances are usually secondary to pain, spasticity, urinary dysfunction, depression, or drug side-effects.

5.1.7 **Sexual dysfunction**

Spinal lesions probably account for the high incidence of erectile dysfunction seen in men with MS, however additional factors such as fatigue, depression, spasticity and anxiety relating to urinary function all contribute to male sexual dysfunction. Sildenafil citrate (a phosphodiesterase type-5 inhibitor; Viagra®) is commonly used to treat erectile dysfunction in MS, although trial data in MS have not been convincing. In women with MS loss of libido and genital sensory changes are common complaints and complications of MS, such as fatigue and depression also play a major role in female sexual dysfunction. Treatments of these associated symptoms may help to improve sexual function.

5.1.8 Gastrointestinal symptoms

Nausea and vomiting is a common accompaniment to acute brainstem lesions. Although usually transient, symptoms can be very distressing. Management is with anti-emetics such as anti-histamines (e.g. cyclizine), dopamine antagonists (e.g. domperidone) and 5-HT_3 receptor antagonists (e.g. ondansetron).

Patients with MS commonly complain of constipation. The aetiology of bowel dysfunction in MS is probably multi-factorial, consisting of a combination of spinal cord dysfunction and generalized systemic factors (drug side effects, generalized immobility). Treatments are geared towards optimizing the mechanics of defaecation through the use of laxatives or irrigation approaches. Constipation is also thought to increase urinary dysfunction in MS, so optimal management may help a number of domains.

5.1.9 Lifestyle advice

Patients with MS often ask about specific lifestyle issues, such as diet or exercise. Although many dietary regimes have been touted as a 'treatment' for MS, no scientific evidence has shown any specific diet to be superior to a standard 'healthy diet'. With increasing interest in vitamin D, patients should be encouraged to eat healthily in order to consume recommended daily amounts of all vitamins. There is no evidence at this time to recommend vitamin supplementation. Similarly with exercise, patients should be encouraged to take regular aerobic exercise in order to maintain cardiovascular fitness. For those patients with disabilities this may be achieved with assistance from a specialist physiotherapist.

With increased access to the internet and the burgeoning of electronic information, patients with MS access information on-line. Although many websites may provide useful information concerning MS, the provision of information on the internet as a whole is not regulated. As such, it is useful to be able to quote a number of reliable websites to patients requiring more information. Typically national MS Society websites are a useful source of information, particularly for the newly-diagnosed. Examples include:

- http://www.mssociety.org.uk
- http://www.nationalmssociety.org
- http://www.mstrust.org.uk.

5.1.10 **Alternative therapies for MS**

Since MS remains incurable and since therapies for the chronic progressive phase are limited, a number of alternative or complimentary therapies have been linked with MS. Whilst many of these therapies are unlikely to worsen MS, the therapeutic effects are unproven. It is likely that many therapies have a placebo effect. Many patients will try therapies such as acupuncture, reflexology, hypnotherapy, and homeopathy. Hyperbaric oxygen therapy has received some attention in relation to MS. This alternative treatment involves breathing oxygen through a mask in a pressurised chamber and is popular with some patients although there is no scientific proof of its efficacy.

5.2 **Modulating disease processes**

Major changes in the way MS is treated have occurred over the past two decades and further improvements in therapies are likely in the future. Disease-modifying therapies are agents which directly attenuate or abrogate some of the pathological processes occurring in MS in order to limit tissue damage. Here, current and 'in-trial' therapies for MS will be discussed.

5.2.1 **Treating relapses**

5.2.1.1 Definition of a relapse

A relapse of MS is defined as an acute 'worsening of function' lasting over 24 hours and accompanied by improvement over the following few weeks (remission). Typically relapses last for several days to weeks before improvement. Frequency of relapses is highly variable in MS patient populations, but figures of one every two years are commonly quoted for the whole MS population. Relapses are commoner early in the natural history of the disease and appear less common once the patient has had the disease for some time. Although relapses are the classic hallmark of the relapsing and remitting phase of the disease, they do occur during progressive disease and should be assessed and treated in the same manner as those occurring in relapsing and remitting disease. Relapses may be triggered by intercurrent infections or stress, and are commoner in the post-partum period than during pregnancy. There is no evidence that common vaccinations trigger relapse.

5.2.1.2 Types of relapse

Relapses are thought to be the physical manifestation of acute inflammatory processes within lesions, causing variable degrees of conduction block, demyelination and axonal injury. Relapses take on many different forms, reflecting the area of the central nervous system affected by the inflammatory process. Remission is thought to occur from resolution of inflammation leading to improved conduction and some degree of remyelination.

Types of relapse include:

- Motor
- Sensory
- Visual
- Brainstem
- Spinal.

5.2.1.3 Differential diagnosis

In assessing patients with suspected relapse several factors should be assessed. It is important to distinguish whether the presenting complaint represents a new symptom. A detailed neurological enquiry relating to the chronology of symptoms and the existing symptoms at the time of suspected relapse is important. Although it is often straightforward to diagnose a relapse with *de novo* symptoms lasting over 24 hours, it can be harder to determine whether severe exacerbations of existing symptoms represent true relapse. Worsening of existing symptoms should prompt a search for infections or systemic illness, which may mimic relapse. In addition the severity and impact of the relapse should be assessed, since these will have important implications concerning the treatment.

5.2.1.4 Investigations

In all patients with suspected MS relapse a detailed neurological history and examination should be performed. The diagnosis of relapse remains a clinical one and brain or spinal cord imaging are not usually required (unless there are atypical features or a suspicion of another pathological process). Baseline observations of temperature, pulse and blood pressure are useful, particularly if steroid therapy is being considered. In addition urine should be analysed for signs of infection since urinary tract infection (UTI) may mimic MS relapse and, furthermore, may significantly worsen if immunosuppressants, such as steroids, are used.

5.2.1.5 Treatment

High-dose corticosteroid treatments remain the mainstay of MS relapse therapy. Steroids have broad anti-inflammatory and immunesuppressant roles, including: reduction in cytokine expression by inflammatory cells; reduction in lymphocyte proliferation; suppression of pro-inflammatory prostaglandins and leukotrienes; reduction in T cell function; and reductions in class II MHC expression on macrophages. Several trials of corticosteroids in MS relapse have been performed which have been the subject of recent Cochrane reviews. Specifically, corticosteroids can be said to improve acute exacerbations of symptoms within the first five weeks and thus improve short-term disability caused by relapse. Meta-analysis of published trials did not show any benefit of steroids on prevention of acute relapses or reduction in long-term disability (although trials concerning this have not been rigorously performed). In addition, short-term (five days) treatments appeared as efficacious as longer treatment protocols.

If MS relapse is suspected and if other causes of neurological deterioration are ruled out, patients with an acute relapse, sufficient to cause distressing symptoms or an increased limitation on activities should be considered for a course of high-dose corticosteroids (see Figure 5.2). Prior to treatment the relative benefits of the treatments versus the potential side-effects should be discussed. The course should be started as soon as possible after onset of the relapse and should be either:

- intravenous methylprednisolone, 500 mg–1 g daily, for between three and five days (typically 1 g daily for three days) or
- high-dose oral methylprednisolone, 500 mg–2 g daily, for between three and five days (typically 500 mg daily for five days).

Usually short courses of steroids are used and it is usually recommended that a course of steroids should last no longer than three weeks. It is generally recommended that steroids should not be given more than three times in any year.

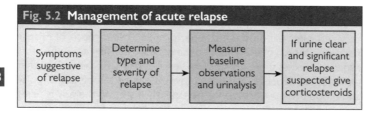

Fig. 5.2 Management of acute relapse

Symptoms suggestive of relapse → Determine type and severity of relapse → Measure baseline observations and urinalysis → If urine clear and significant relapse suspected give corticosteroids

Whether oral or intravenous steroids are more efficacious in acute relapse is often debated. Individual trials and meta-analyses of trials have supported the notion that there is no significant difference in clinical or radiological outcome following oral compared to intravenous therapy. Issues such as convenience, access to services and the patient's own preferences should be taken into account when prescribing steroids.

High-dose steroids have potential side effects which should be discussed with patients prior to commencing treatments. Chronic administration of steroids in MS is not recommended, thus reducing the risk of side effects induced by chronic steroid administration, such as osteoporosis, hypertension, and diabetes. Potential side effects of short-term high dose steroid administration are listed. Side effects usually improve on cessation of therapy.

> **Box 5.1 Potential side effects of a short course of high dose steroids**
>
> **Side effect**
>
> - Alteration in mood, either with euphoria or depression
> - Insomnia
> - Gastrointestinal symptoms, commonly dyspepsia (patients are often co-prescribed proton pump inhibitors e.g. lansoprazole)
> - Increased appetite
> - Flushing
> - Palpitations
> - Acne
> - Ankle swelling
> - Very rarely: avascular necrosis of the hip.

Often patients enquire whether they should continue with physiotherapy during a relapse. There is no evidence to suggest that physical exercise worsens relapses, although Uhtoff's phenomenon may lead to exacerbation of symptoms during exercise. There is some evidence to suggest that a combination of steroid therapy and physiotherapy may speed up recovery from relapse.

5.2.1.6 Implication of relapses for further treatments
Currently licensed disease-modifying therapies reduce relapse rates. Thus awareness of individual relapse rates is important when considering these therapies. Patients with high relapse rates are more likely to benefit from these medications and these issues should be discussed at or shortly after the time of relapse.

5.2.2 **Preventing relapses**
A major drive in recent years has been to develop agents that will reduce symptomatic relapses. Two major drug classes have been in routine clinical use for a number of years: beta interferons (βIFN) and glatiramer acetate (GA). In addition the monoclonal antibody natalizumab has been licensed for use in severe disease, and several therapies are in trial.

5.2.2.1 Disease-modifying therapies in MS
Ideally a disease-modifying therapy (DMT) in MS would:

- Reduce ongoing symptoms
- Reduce number of relapses
- Reduce disease progression.

At present the currently licensed DMTs have been shown to have effects predominantly on numbers of relapses. Their effects on reduction in disease progression are still being investigated. It is hoped that some of the newer drug therapies combined with earlier treatment regimes will reduce the number of patients entering into the secondary progressive phase of the disease.

The βIFNs and GA are the most widely used DMTs for MS. Due to their broadly similar efficacy and similar modes of administration they are often considered together. Decisions on which to choose depend on several factors including frequency of administration, mode of administration and potential side-effects. The major DMTs are shown in Table 5.3:

Table 5.3 **Characteristics of commonly used DMTs**				
	Avonex®	**Betaferon®**	**Rebif®**	**Copaxone®**
Active molecule	βIFN-1a	βIFN-1b	βIFN-1a	Glatiramer acetate
Dose and frequency	30 mcg once weekly	300 mcg alternate days	22–44 mcg three times per week	20 mg daily
Mode of administration	intra-muscular	sub-cutaneous	sub-cutaneous	sub-cutaneous

5.2.2.2 βIFN

Three major βIFNs have been in clinical use for a number of years: Avonex® (βIFN-1a); Rebif® (βIFN-1a); Betaferon® (βIFN-1b; Betaseron®). A further form of βIFN-1b was marketed in 2009 as Extavia. They differ in their mode and frequency of administration with Avonex® being given the least frequently but having to be given by the more painful intra-muscular route.

Mechanisms of action of βIFNs are not fully understood and are likely to involve a number of mechanisms.

Box 5.2 Mechanism of action of βIFN

- Mechanisms of clinical efficacy still not entirely understood
- Thought that β-interferons have general anti-inflammatory effects
- Studies have also suggested that β-interferon has effects on reducing traffic of immune cells through the impaired blood brain barrier in the disease
- Other theories include inhibition of T-cell activation and proliferation; apoptosis of autoreactive T cells; induction of regulatory T cells; cytokine modulation; and potential antiviral action
- Most of the effects studied either in vitro or in animal models of the disease, and although immune effects are observed in humans taking β-interferon, the precise mode of action in MS is unknown.

Early pivotal trials of βIFNs have indicated a modest reduction in annualized relapse rates of all three major drugs by roughly one third. Trials have indicated probable equivalence of efficacy of the three major βIFNS (and GA). They do not appear to prevent or slow disease progression.

MRI data have been extensively collected from patients enrolled in treatment trials. All licensed drugs have shown early reductions in MRI activity (using T2 lesion volume or gadolinium enhancing lesions) compared to placebo control. The clinical relevance of this change has been questioned.

Side effects are common with βIFNS. Many patients experience 'flu-like symptoms often occurring shortly after injection. These symptoms usually respond to non-steroidal anti-inflammatory drugs or anti-pyretics, but in around 10% of patients they may be severe enough to cause them to discontinue the drugs. Other side effects include depression and injection-site reactions.

5.2.2.3 Glatiramer acetate (GA)
GA was developed following observations in animal models of central nervous system inflammation. Its mechanisms of action remain poorly understood, but possibly involve a number of mechanisms.

Box 5.3 Mechanism of action of GA

- GA is a random sequence polypeptide (composed of four amino acids that are found in myelin basic protein)
- Initially developed as an agent to induce experimental autoimmune encephalomyelitis in mice, but found to be protective against this condition
- Mode of action uncertain
- Reduction in relapses may occur by causing competition with myelin antigens for binding to MHC class II molecules and thus a reduction in myelin damage
- More likely GA works by inducing tolerance or anergy of myelin-reactive lymphocytes.

In a similar manner to βIFNs, it has been shown to reduce the annualised relapse rates by approximately one third compared to placebo. Again, there seems to be no useful impact on disease progression.

The commonest side effect of GA is an injection site reaction, which in some cases can be extensive.

5.2.2.4 Starting βIFN or GA
When deciding to start DMTs the risk benefit ratios of the drugs must be presented. Since the drugs offer no cure and only modest benefits, and since the drugs are not administered orally, a frank discussion concerning their potential use should be conducted with

the patient. In other words, do the beneficial effects of the drug outweigh the potential side effects or difficulties administering the drug? If a patient has not had recent significant relapses, trial data would suggest they would not benefit from DMTs.

In view of these difficulties, guidelines have been drawn up to aid the decision process for starting DMTs. In the UK, the Association of British Neurologists has suggested that:

- Patients with **RRMS** should be offered DMTs if they:
  - are able to walk over 100m without assistance
  - have had at least two disabling relapses in the last two years
  - are aged over 18 and have no contra-indications to the drugs
- Patients with **SPMS** should be offered DMTs if they:
  - are able to walk over 10 m without assistance
  - have had at least two disabling relapses in the last two years
  - have had minimal increase in disability over the past two years
  - they are aged over 18 and have no contra-indications to the drugs.

It is important to provide patients with information concerning the nature of the DMTs and realistic expectations of what the drugs will achieve. This should be done in conjunction with MS nurses who are able to show the injection devices used and discuss the practicalities of treatments. The drugs are not recommended during pregnancy.

Some clinicians advocate starting DMTs at presentation with a clinically isolated syndrome (CIS). Trial data has shown that DMTs reduce the conversion rate of CIS to clinically definite MS from 45–50% with placebo to 28–35% with interferon over the 2–3 years of the trials, though this is likely a delay rather than any more profound interference with the disease. There is no good evidence of an effect on disability rates that is gained by early treatment. Decisions on treatment in CIS are difficult due to the problems predicting disease course at onset and must always take into account issues such as treatment tolerability, mode of administration and likely benefit.

Since these DMTs have roughly equal efficacy, the decision concerning which agent to commence is often made on the basis of convenience and acceptability of a particular drug to the individual patient.

5.2.2.5 Stopping or switching βIFN and GA

There are several reasons to consider stopping DMTs including side effects of the drugs, inconvenience of use, and failure of therapy. An algorithm for decisions relating to problems encountered with the drugs is given (see Figure 5.3).

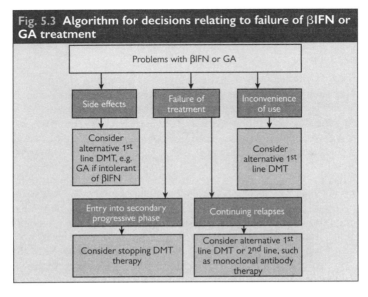

Fig. 5.3 Algorithm for decisions relating to failure of βIFN or GA treatment

Problems with βIFN or GA

Side effects

Failure of treatment

Inconvenience of use

Consider alternative 1st line DMT, e.g. GA if intolerant of βIFN

Consider alternative 1st line DMT

Entry into secondary progressive phase

Continuing relapses

Consider stopping DMT therapy

Consider alternative 1st line DMT or 2nd line, such as monoclonal antibody therapy

If a patient is intolerant of a particular therapy, it is usually advisable to try a different agent, e.g. if problematic side effects are encountered with βIFN the patient may wish to use GA. Similarly if the mode or frequency of administration is not tolerated, a different drug or formulation may be used. Women wishing to become pregnant should ideally come off the drugs prior to conception.

Decisions relating to poor efficacy of βIFN or GA may be more difficult. If a patient is clearly experiencing progressive neurological disability, in the absence of clinical relapses, it is sensible to discuss cessation of treatment, since the drugs are not efficacious for preventing secondary disability. However, if relapses are occurring despite βIFN or GA therapy, patients should be considered for second-line drugs, such as natalizumab.

5.2.2.6 βIFNS and GA and long-term disability

Many of the early trials were short (two to three years) and were not able to answer whether treatment with βIFN or GA had any effects on long-term disability. The chronic nature of the disease and slowness of disease progression makes studies very difficult to perform or interpret. Longer studies and follow-up data have suggested βIFN or GA may reduce time to entry into secondary progression. However, it is thought (from epidemiological data) that once secondary progression has commenced, suppression of inflammation is unlikely to impact on further disease progression. Intuitively, reduction in relapses would seem likely to reduce long-term disability, but conclusive evidence that βIFN or GA reduce long-term disability is still lacking. βIFN or GA have not been shown to have efficacy in secondary progressive MS or primary progressive MS and are not recommended for use in these circumstances, unless the patient is experiencing significant relapses.

5.2.2.7 Natalizumab

Natalizumab (trade name: Tysabri®) is a humanized monoclonal antibody (IgG4) directed against the very late antigen-4 (VLA-4) adhesion molecule present on the surface of lymphocytes and monocytes. It is thought to exert its effects via blocking of VLA-4, thus preventing its interaction with VCAM-1 (vascular cell adhesion molecule-1), a process which is important in the trafficking of inflammatory cells across the blood brain barrier. In clinical trials, natalizumab has been shown to reduce risk of relapse by 68% compared to placebo or when used in combination with Avonex® has been shown to reduce risk of relapse by 56% compared to Avonex® alone. Reductions in the risk of sustained accumulated disability have also been shown with the drug. A major issue, however, with the use of the drug have been rare incidences of progressive multifocal leucoencephalopathy (PML) following treatment. The incidence of PML with natalizumab seems to be in the order of 1 in 2,000 patients.

Natalizumab is given as a monthly intravenous infusion and is currently recommended for use in patients with early aggressive multiple sclerosis. It may also be considered in patients who continue to relapse despite βIFN or GA therapy. Other than PML, side effects include allergic reactions to the drug (4%) and abnormalities in liver function, with occasional reports of liver damage. Monitoring of the drug includes serial liver function tests and awareness of the possibility of PML. A rapid deterioration or unusual symptoms should prompt urgent imaging. Many authorities recommend treatment withdrawal after a fixed period, as the risk of PML appears to be related the duration of therapy. A recrudescence of disease activity can, however, accompany natalizumab withdrawal.

5.2.2.8 Mitoxantrone

Mitoxantrone is a topoisomerase II inhibitor which disrupts DNA within cells and limits DNA repair. It is used as a chemotherapeutic agent for a number of cancers. It is a powerful immunosuppressive agent which crosses the blood brain barrier and in experimental models of MS has multiple immune-modulating effects. It is sometimes used for rapidly evolving multiple sclerosis or severe progressive relapsing disease. In many centres it is used as a second line 'rescue therapy' for patients who have not responded well to βIFN or GA. Clinical trials have suggested that mitoxantrone may reduce annualized relapse rates by 60–70%.

Mitoxantrone is administered via intravenous infusion. The main limitations to its use are its potential risks and side effects. The most serious risks are the long-term potential of cardiotoxicity and leukaemia. Regarding cardiotoxicity, pre-treatment echocardiography should be performed, with careful monitoring of left ventricular ejection fraction (LVEF) before each cycle of treatment. If 10% reduction in LVEF or LVEF less than 50% is documented, the treatment should be discontinued. Therapy related acute leukaemia occurs in up to 3 per 1,000 of MS patients treated with mitoxantrone and careful monitoring is required. Less severe side effects include nausea and vomiting, alopecia and amenorrhoea.

5.2.2.9 Fingolimod
This sphingosine-1-phosphate agonist is thought to act by preventing lymphocyte migration into the central nervous system. Fingolimod is an oral agent and trials have shown >50% reduction in annualized relapse rates. It has recently been approved for use in the USA and Europe and is the first licensed oral agent for disease modification in MS. Serious reported adverse effects include bradycardia and skin cancers.

5.2.2.10 Drugs in trial
A number of newer therapeutic agents are currently in trial or in the early stages of licensing. These include:

- *Alemtuzumab*: this humanized monoclonal antibody targets CD52, a protein found on lymphocytes and monocytes. Formerly known as CAMPATH-1H, treatment with the drug induces profound lymphopaenia. It is used for the treatment of chronic lymphocytic leukaemia and a number of other autoimmune diseases. In MS, it is highly efficacious in suppressing relapses. In a recent trial comparing to βIFN (Rebif®), alemtuzumab reduced the risk of relapse and risk of sustained accumulation of disability by >70% compared to βIFN. The main concerns over treatment have been the emergence of other autoimmune diseases, typically thyroid autoimmunity. Further trials are on-going

- *Daclizumab*: this humanized IgG1 monoclonal antibody binds to the interleukin-2 receptor (α-chain), thus limiting maturation and expansion of activated T cells. Again, it appears highly effective in reducing disease activity (reducing gadolinium enhancing lesions on MRI scan). Long-term data concerning safety and efficacy are, however, still awaited

- *Rituximab*: this monoclonal antibody therapy targets CD20 present on B cells and induces their cytolysis. It is used for a number of conditions, including rheumatoid arthritis. The humanised successor of rituximab, ocrelizumab, is currently in trial

- *Cladribine*: this is a further potential oral agent. It is an adenosine deaminase-resistant nucleoside analogue which induces selective lymphotoxicity. Trials have shown approximately 60% reduction in annualized relapse rates compared to placebo. However, safety concerns, particularly induction of cancers, has led to the rejection of cladribine by the majority of national drug regulatory bodies and the subsequent withdrawal of the drug (for MS indications) by its manufacturers.

Suggested reading

Burton, J.M., et al. (2009) Oral versus intravenous steroids for treatment of relapses in multiple sclerosis. *Cochrane Database Syst Rev*, **2009**(3): CD006921.

Filippini, G., et al. (2004) Corticosteroids or ACTH for acute exacerbations in multiple sclerosis. *Cochrane Database Syst Rev* **2000**(4): p. CD001331.

Fowler, C.J., et al. (2009) A UK consensus on the management of the bladder in multiple sclerosis. *Postgrad Med J*, **85**(1008): 552–9.

IFNB Multiple Sclerosis Study Group (1993) Interferon beta-1b is effective in relapsing-remitting multiple sclerosis. I. Clinical results of a multicenter, randomized, double-blind, placebo-controlled trial. *Neurology* **43**(4): 655–61.

Jacobs, L.D., et al. (1996) Intramuscular interferon beta-1a for disease progression in relapsing multiple sclerosis. The Multiple Sclerosis Collaborative Research Group (MSCRG). *Ann Neurol*, **39**(3): 285–94.

Johnson, K.P., et al. (1995) Copolymer 1 reduces relapse rate and improves disability in relapsing-remitting multiple sclerosis: results of a phase III multicenter, double-blind placebo-controlled trial. The Copolymer 1 Multiple Sclerosis Study Group. *Neurology*, **45**(7): 1268–76.

PRISMS (Prevention of Relapses and Disability by Interferon beta-1a Subcutaneously in Multiple Sclerosis) Study Group (1998) Randomised double-blind placebo-controlled study of interferon beta-1a in relapsing/remitting multiple sclerosis. *Lancet* **352**(9139): 1498–504.

Chapter 6

Future avenues for research in multiple sclerosis

Key points

- Better understanding of the causes of MS will lead to better therapies for the disease
- Understanding why disease phenotypes are so variable and identifying prognostic factors which will predict the early disease course will help to develop better therapeutic protocols
- Future therapies will need to be targeted at reducing progressive disability.

Despite the significant advances in understanding and treating MS, many aspects of our understanding of the disease remain incomplete. A number of unanswered questions remain, the answers to which will, over time, provide improved prospects for those diagnosed with the illness.

In this chapter, we will briefly review some of those questions and postulate future avenues for advancement of knowledge in the disease.

6.1 What causes MS?

This remains one of the commonest questions that newly diagnosed patients will ask during clinic consultations and it is one to which no easy answer can be given. Most would now agree that MS is a complex disorder which occurs in those with some degree of genetic susceptibility. A number of environmental factors may act in concord or separately to provide the disease phenotype. The lack of a specific aetiological factor has been the major reason that no strategy has been instituted to prevent the disease or reduce its incidence.

In the future, we may have a better understanding of how susceptible genotypes may interact with environmental triggers to cause disease. It is possible, therefore, that in years to come specific disease-modifying or even disease-preventing therapies may be implemented for specific genotypes. For instance, it may be that a viral trigger (e.g. EBV) leads to the disease only on the background of susceptible genotypes and those people with an 'at-risk' genotype may benefit from anti-viral therapies. In a similar way, further understanding of the genetic basis for the disease may lead to the advancement of other pharmacogenetic strategies and individualized disease-modifying therapies.

6.2 **Can MS be diagnosed at an earlier stage in its natural history (and will that help)?**

Because of the development of a number of disease-modifying therapies in recent years, there has been a drive to develop protocols for earlier diagnosis of MS. Classically the diagnosis has depended on at least two clinical episodes occurring at different time points. Based on the assumption that institution of therapy should start at the earliest possible time, criteria have been developed for earlier diagnosis of the disease centred on paraclinical evidence of disease activity. Most notably, the McDonald criteria have been used in a large number of studies and have 'allowed' diagnosis of MS based on one clinical episode (CIS) with subsequent radiological evidence of dissemination of the disease in time and space. Whilst this approach has been informative in studying the natural history of MS and in developing approaches to therapy for CIS, a significant number of people with 'McDonald criteria MS' may not go on to have further clinical events. The challenge of natural history studies and diagnostic criteria of the future will be to pick out those at high risk of aggressive disease who require early treatment and those who will have relatively benign disease who would not require early aggressive therapies.

6.3 **How can we better understand the natural history of the disease and why is the phenotype so variable?**

One of the most fascinating and yet inexplicable aspects of MS is the variability in disease phenotype. Between 10–15% of patients will have a benign course, whereas others will have more rapidly progressive disease and an aggressive phenotype. Trying to predict which disease course an individual patient will follow at presentation is very difficult but important; firstly to try and give the individual some idea about disease prognosis and, secondly, to plan for therapies. In someone whose disease course is going to be relatively benign treatment with aggressive immunosuppression would not be in the patient's best interest; whereas someone with early aggressive disease should be considered for such treatment. In future years, the development of better biomarkers (either imaging or biological samples) to predict early disease course and future prognosis will be a major drive, so disease-modifying therapies can be directed appropriately. In a related manner, understanding disease mechanisms which underpin tissue damage will help to tailor specific therapies for specific aspects of the disease. The separation of neuromyelitis optica from MS and the discovery of the anti-aquaporin-4 antibody in the disorder have directed therapies to address antibody-mediated tissue injury. Similarly, addressing neurodegenerative aspects of secondary progressive disease will, hopefully, reduce the burden of chronic disability.

6.4 **What future therapies will be available?**

There have been significant advances in treating MS. However, certain aspects of the disease remain poorly treated. Notably, once patients have entered the progressive phase of the disease (either progressive from outset (PPMS) or secondary progressive) there is little in the way of effective therapy that will significantly reduce further disability. Since relapses in MS can be reduced by a number of therapies it has been postulated that early and aggressive treatment of relapses before disease progression has set in may prevent entry into the secondary progressive phase of the disease. Whether this holds true and how early is early are the subject of current trials. The hope remains, however, that decline into disease progression may be terminated in a significant number of people by early aggressive therapy. Even if this strategy proves effective, there are likely to be patients who enter the secondary progressive phase (either because they are progressive from outset or the therapies have been instituted too late). For those, treatment of disease progression is required. The pathological substrate for disease progression appears to be predominantly axonal degeneration and so therapies to protect axons specifically will be needed. The concept of neuroprotection is well recognized in other neurodegenerative disorders and is becoming increasingly studied in relation to MS. A major issue concerning trials in progressive disease is the problem of measuring disability and the inherent difficulties of studying a slowly deteriorating condition. The trials of disease-modifying therapies which have formed the basis for current therapies have predominantly used relapses (as a defined clinical entity) as the outcome measure. Many trials use disability scores, such as EDSS, as a measure of disability although such measures have problems and limitations. In future design of therapies for disease progression need to be improved and more reproducible measures of disability need to be assessed.

Stem cells have attracted interest in all fields of regenerative medicine. Trials are ongoing in MS and have mostly focused on bone marrow cell therapies, either as a strategy to 're-boot' the immune system and thus reduce the level of autoimmunity, to provide general anti-inflammatory function or to provide general trophic support to the diseased nervous system. Such therapies may hold much hope for future generations.

Suggested reading

Polman, C.H., et al. (2005) Diagnostic criteria for multiple sclerosis: 2005 revisions to the 'McDonald Criteria'. *Ann Neurol* **58**(6): 840–6.

Wilkins, A. and Scolding, N. (2008) Protecting axons in multiple sclerosis. *Mult Scler* **14**(8): 1013–25.

Chapter 7

Childhood onset multiple sclerosis

> **Key points**
> - MS is uncommon in paediatric populations
> - The differential diagnosis of MS in children differs from that in adults
> - The principles of treatment in childhood onset MS are similar to those in adults, although trial-evidence base for treatments in children is lacking.

MS is a rare disease of childhood which may be difficult to distinguish from other paediatric demyelinating conditions. Approximately 5% of all cases of MS occur in childhood (under age of 18). When the disease occurs in the very young whose brain is still developing, the manifestations may be different to adult disease.

This chapter will focus on summarizing the epidemiology of childhood MS; information concerning possible aetiologies derived from the study of childhood MS; specific presenting complaints; the differential diagnosis; and treatments.

7.1 Epidemiology of childhood MS

A recent Canadian study determined the incidence of all acquired demyelinating conditions of childhood, including acute disseminated encephalomyelitis (ADEM), transverse myelitis (TM), optic neuritis and MS to be 0.9 per 100,000 in that country. Although approximately 5% of all cases of MS are diagnosed before the age of 18, up to 10% may experience their first relapse of MS during childhood. Most children with MS experience their first relapse of the disease between the ages of 9 and 13. Studies on the sex ratios of paediatric MS are not complete, but the female:male ratio is probably of the order of 3:1.

The role of ethnicity in childhood MS has attracted some attention. The typical ethnic patterns seen in adult MS patients are generally less observable in children with the disease and indeed some studies report a higher incidence of Caribbean, Middle Eastern and Asian ancestry in childhood cases than of Northern European ancestry.

Because of the relative rarity of the disorder in children and some of the difficulties of diagnosing the illness, the epidemiology of childhood MS is not as well defined as that in adult populations.

7.2 **Causes of childhood MS**

The potential aetiological factors in adult MS have been discussed in Chapter 2. The link between EBV and MS is stronger in paediatric populations and it has been estimated that EBV positivity increases the risk of MS by roughly threefold. There is evidence specifically linking the EBV nuclear antigen 1 (EBNA1) since high titres are often found in childhood MS. Discovering infectious factors that may trigger MS may be easier to determine in children, since the time between infection and neurological disease is shorter and children are likely to have been infected with fewer infectious agents at the time of presentation. Interestingly one study has suggested a lower rate of chicken pox (varicella zoster) infection in children with MS compared to control populations.

Migration studies in MS have been particularly informative. The conclusion from many of these studies is that children who migrate before adolescence appear to adopt more closely the risk of their adopted country (albeit that they may present during adulthood). This compares to those who migrate later who keep the risk more associated with their country of origin. This may imply that environmental factors acting in a specific 'at risk' period of youth unlocks disease susceptibility.

Other general factors involved in disease aetiology and susceptibility are discussed in Chapter 2.

7.3 **Presenting features of childhood MS**

In keeping with adult-onset MS, children may present in a number of ways. Since the differential diagnosis of an acute demyelinating disorders in children is wide and differs from adults in the relative likelihood of other diagnoses, careful history taking and examination, coupled with diagnostic investigations, are required. As with adult populations, the diagnosis of MS requires evidence of clinical (or radiological) evidence of dissemination of disease in time and space. Although patients may present with their first clinical event during childhood, the diagnosis of MS is often made in adulthood.

Presentation of childhood MS include:

- *Optic Neuritis*: Up to one-third of children with MS present with optic neuritis (ON). In young children symptoms of ON may be difficult to ascertain. ON causes reduced vision (particularly colour perception) often with pain on ocular movement. The examination of children with suspected ON can be difficult but may show an increased central scotoma with reduced ability to perform Ishihara charts. ON may occur in the context of ADEM. The differential diagnosis of ON in children includes Leber's Hereditary Optic Neuropathy (LHON), neuromyelitis optica (NMO) spectrum or other inflammatory or ischaemic optic neuropathies.

- *Transverse myelitis*: Approximately 10% of children with MS present with transverse myelitis (TM). Patients present with a subacute (usually evolving over a few days) spinal cord syndrome. In keeping with adult causes of TM, the differential is wide. Again ADEM and neuromyelitis optica spectrum disorders should be considered. In addition, structural lesions, ischaemia, infection, and connective tissue disorders are differential diagnoses. Investigations are particularly helpful, particularly MRI scanning of the spinal cord. The presence of longitudinally extensive transverse myelitis (LETM); extending over more than three vertebral segments) on spinal MRI is suggestive of NMO.

- *Other presentations*: Children may present with their first demyelinating episode in a variety of other manners. Cerebellar and sensory episodes are also common. Studies on paediatric presentations of MS suggest that polysymptomatic presentation may be commoner than in adult groups. Cognitive deficits in the form of subacute encephalopathy have been reported in paediatric MS, although in such cases ADEM should be strongly considered.

7.4 **Diagnosis and differential diagnosis**

The differential diagnosis depends on the clinical course and is helped by MRI appearances. The primary progressive phenotype of MS is very rare in children and progressive neurological decline in children with white matter lesions should prompt a search for alternative diagnoses. The differential diagnosis of acute or subacute demyelinating disorders in children differs from that of adult populations in terms of disease frequencies. However, investigations of suspected demyelination in children follow similar lines to those in adults with additional considerations. MRI imaging, spinal fluid analysis and evoked potentials are routinely used.

Differential diagnoses are summarized in Figure 7.1.

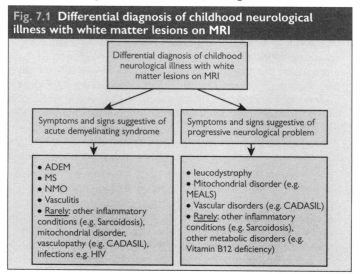

Fig. 7.1 Differential diagnosis of childhood neurological illness with white matter lesions on MRI

Differential diagnoses of acute demyelinating syndromes in children include:

ADEM: Acute disseminated encephalomyelitis (ADEM) is an acute illness characterized by multifocal neurological symptoms and signs with encephalopathy, often with an antecedent history of an acute viral illness. It is usually monophasic, occurs more commonly in children than in adults and the majority of children make a good recovery. Children usually present with an encephalopathic illness, which ranges from behavioural change to drowsiness and coma. The presentation may be similar to the first presentation of MS (clinically isolated syndrome) and it may be difficult to determine whether the illness represents an acute monophasic illness or the first presentation of MS. The encephalopathy of ADEM may be the most useful clinical pointer in distinguishing it from CIS. MRI appearances may help to distinguish ADEM from MS and oligoclonal bands are usually absent in the CSF of ADEM patients (see Figure 7.2).

Neuromyelitis optica: Neuromyelitis optica is characterized by the presence of transverse myelitis with optic neuritis, with additional features of LETM; absence of brain MRI lesions; and NMO IgG seropositivity (see Chapter 3).

CNS vasculitis: CNS vasculitis presents with fevers, headache, cognitive changes, seizures and other focal neurological signs. MRI often reveals multifocal white and grey matter changes and may be similar to ADEM or MS. Brain biopsy is often required to make a definitive diagnosis, since angiography may not detect all cases.

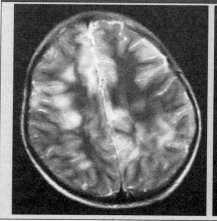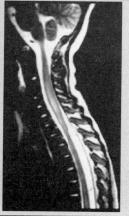

Fig. 7.2 **MRI scan of brain and cervical spine of a 10 year old child with ADEM; scans kindly provided by Dr. Shelley Renowden, Neuroradiologist, Frenchay Hospital, Bristol, UK**

Differential diagnoses of progressive neurological deterioration in children with white matter lesions include:

Leucodystrophies: these are a group of disorders causing white matter damage. The commonest is adrenoleukodystrophy (ALD) which is X-linked and caused by a mutation in a peroxisomal gene. The disease typically presents in boys with progressive neurological decline in childhood with or without adrenal disease. Some males present later with adrenomyeloneuropathy. Females may be carriers of the disease and may manifest as an MS-like illness in adulthood. Thus a family history of 'MS' in children with a neurological disorder should prompt the search for ALD. Serum very long chain fatty acids (VLCFAs) are typically elevated in ALD.

Mitochondrial disorders: Two main mitochondrial disease phenotypes may mimic MS. Leber's Hereditary Optic Neuropathy (LHON) typically presents with bilateral or sequential optic neuritis with poor recovery of vision. Other symptoms and signs may be present and white matter lesions similar to those seen in MS may be demonstrated on MRI. Specific mitochondrial DNA mutations can be tested to diagnose LHON. Mitochondrial encephalopathy, lactic acidosis and stroke-like episodes (MELAS) is typically maternally inherited and the phenotype may be caused by mutations in a number of mitochondrial genes. Its presentation may be similar to ADEM or MS. As with LHON, specific mitochondrial DNA mutations are tested in order to make the diagnosis.

7.5 Treatment of paediatric MS

Treatment of paediatric MS is based upon studies performed in patients with adult-onset disease (see Chapter 5). Due to the nature and rarity of the disorders in children definitive studies on efficacy of disease modifying therapies are lacking. Several small studies of βIFN have been performed on paediatric populations which suggest the reduction in annualized relapse rates seen in adult populations are probably similar in children. If a child fails treatment on a first-line therapy (βIFN or glatiramer actate), decisions on second line therapy may be difficult and long term risks of some of the more potent immunosuppressants need to be considered. Again there is very little evidence from studies in children concerning the optimal second-line disease modifying therapy.

Suggested reading

Ghezzi, A., et al. (2010) The management of multiple sclerosis in children: a European view. *Mult Scler* **16**(10): 1258–67.

Venkateswaran, S. and Banwell, B. (2010) Pediatric multiple sclerosis. *Neurologist* **16**(2): 92–105.

Yeh, E.A., et al. (2009) Pediatric multiple sclerosis. *Nat Rev Neurol* **5**(11): 621–31.

Index